Vegan

Recipes

Table of Contents

CRISPY VEGAN QUINOA CAKES WITH TOMATO-CHICKPEA RELISH

Crispy Vegan Quinoa Cakes (with no eggs, flour or bread crumbs) topped with Tomato Chickpea Relish- a healthy flavorful, plant-based VEGAN dinner that is delicious and gluten-free! It can be made ahead!

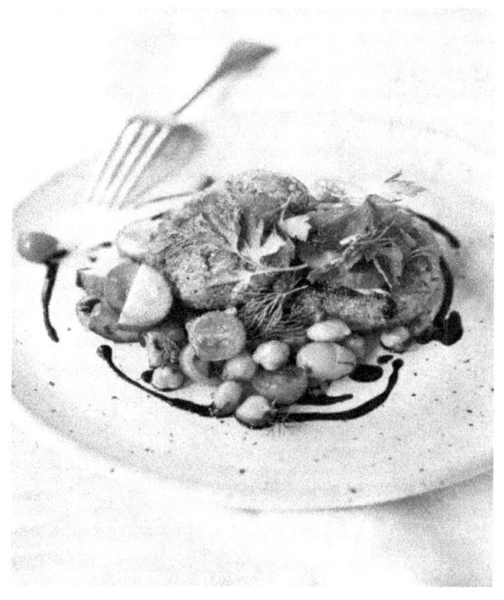

Prep Time:	Total Time:	Cook Time	Amount Per Serving
45 minutes	1 hour 15 minutes	30	Serves 4

Description

Crispy Vegan Quinoa Cakes with Tomato Chickpea Relish- a delicious, healthy, flavorful plant-based vegan dinner that is gluten-free. Please watch the how-to video to see how to get the quinoa to "clump".

Method: Stove Top

Ingredients

Quinoa Cakes (use white quinoa – tri-colored, or other colored quinoa will not bind)

- 2 cups water
- 1 cup rinsed, white quinoa (rinse and drain!!! DON'T SKIP)
- 2 teaspoons olive oil
- 1 tsp cumin
- 1 teaspoon granulated garlic powder
- 1/2 tsp kosher salt
- 1/2 teaspoon herbs de Provence (or Italian dried herbs)
- zest from one small lemon (optional)
- 1/4 cup chopped Italian parsley (optional)
- Fresh Tomato Chickpea Relish
- 2 cups cherry or grape tomatoes, sliced in half
- 1 cup cucumber, diced
- 1/4 cup fresh basil (or flat-leaf parsley, dill, or mint, or a combo!) chopped
- 1/4 cup chopped scallions (or finely sliced red onion)
- 1 ½ cup cooked chickpeas (1 can, drained and rinsed)
- 3 Tbs olive oil
- 3 Tbs balsamic vinegar
- 1/4 tsp salt… more to taste
- 1 small minced garlic clove (optional)

Optional Garnishes: Crumbled Goat Cheese, balsamic glaze

Instructions

In a medium pot, over high heat, add rinsed white quinoa, salt, garlic powder, cumin, dried herbs, olive oil, and stir. Bring to a boil. Cover, lower heat to low, and simmer gently for 20 minutes. Set timer.

While the quinoa is cooking make the Tomato Chickpea Relish, stirring all ingredients together in a medium bowl.

Check quinoa- making sure all the water is gone. If not, continue cooking covered, 5 more minutes, and until steam holes appear (this usually takes me a total of 25 minutes) and quinoa has soaked up all the water and looks fairly dry.) It is important that quinoa is dry-ish and not watery. Be patient here, all stoves are different.

While it's still warm, stir the quinoa vigorously with a fork, for a one whole minute, until you begin to see the individual grains break apart. This is imperative, to getting the quinoa to bind. Eventually, after a full minute of stirring, the grains will break apart and begin to clump. You can visually see this. Remove from stove, let cool down in the pot to where it's cool enough to handle with your hands, about 15 minutes. Stir in the lemon zest and fresh parsley if you like.

Using wet hands, shape into 4 balls, the size of a tennis ball. Place on a plate or sheet pan. Using wet hands press into a 1 – 1 1/2 inch thick cake (about 3-4 inches wide), smoothing any cracks on the edges, and making them nice and tidy. Wet hands is key.

Refrigerate 15 minutes to set. As the quinoa cakes cool they will become even sturdier. (These will keep 3-4 days if made ahead, just lightly oil them, cover, and store in the fridge.)

Gently Pan-sear the Quinoa Cakes in a well-oiled skillet (using a thin metal spatula to flip) over medium heat. You can pan-sear them without any coating, or for an extra crispy crust, dredge in rice flour or GF Panko. I often do these without any coating at all. Just be sure to not fiddle with them- letting them develop a good crust before flipping. As then develop the crust, they will naturally release themselves from the pan. I like to use a thin metal spatula to flip (more precise).

You can also bake these in a toaster oven (right on the rack) or in a 400F oven (on a parchment-lined pan) until warmed through, about 20 minutes, but the crust for a skillet gives these the BEST texture.

Divide among plates and top with the fresh tomato chickpea relish. Spoon any remaining dressing over top and around the cakes.

CHIPOTLE PORTOBELLO TACOS (VEGAN!)

These Vegan Portobello Tacos are full of flavor! Made with sheet-pan roasted Portobello mushrooms in a delicious chipotle marinade, with vegan Cilantro Cream, avocado, pickled onions, and roasted peppers. Smoky, spicy and "meaty' these vegan tacos are hearty and delicious!

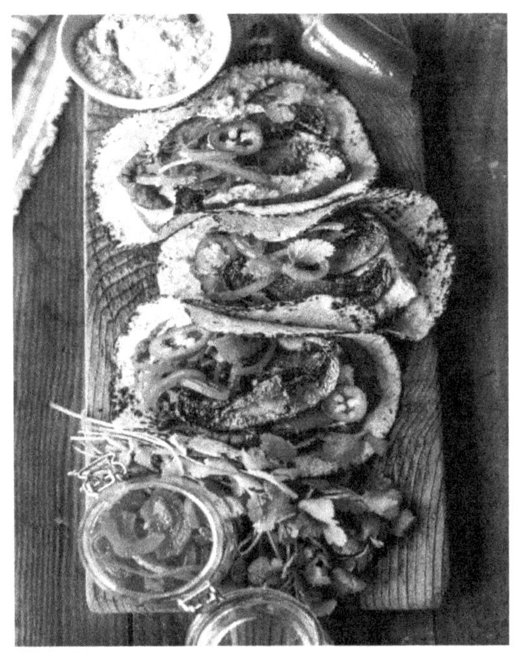

Prep Time	Total Time	Cook Time	Amount Per Serving
10	30 minutes	20	Serves 3

Cuisine	**Mediterranean**
Category	Vegan main, dinner

Description

Sheet-Pan, Chipotle Portobello Tacos – smoky, spicy and "meaty" – these VEGAN tacos are sure to satisfy even the most diehard meat-lovers!

Method: Oven Roasted

Ingredients

- 2 extra-large Portobello mushrooms
- 1 red bell pepper
- 1/2 an onion – optional Chipotle Marindade
- 1 tablespoon oil
- 2 tablespoons canned Chipotle in Adobo sauce (SAUCE ONLY)
- 1 minced garlic clove (or ½ teaspoon granulated garlic)
- 1/2 teaspoon cumin
- 1/2 teaspoon coriander salt to taste
- 4 tortillas, warmed
- 1 can refried black beans, warmed

Optional Garnishes: cilantro, pickled onions, Vegan Cilantro Crema or guacamole or sliced avocado.

Instructions

Preheat oven to 425F

Slice the portobellos into ½ inch thick wedges and slice bell pepper in to ½ thick strips. If adding onion, cut into ½ inch thick rings or half-moons.

Place all on a sheet-pan lined sheet pan & Mix marinade ingredients together in a small bowl.

Brush both sides of mushrooms liberally with the marinade, then remaining red bell pepper and onion lightly. Sprinkle portobellos with salt. Roast 20 minutes or until portobellos are fork-tender.

While this is roasting, heat the beans any prep any additional garnishes. Pickled onions and Vegan cilantro Crema both take about 10 minutes to make. Or simply use avocado slices.

When ready to serve, warm the tortillas (over a gas flame on the stove, or in a toaster oven) and spread generously with the refried black beans. Divide chipotle portobellos and peppers (and onions if used) among the tortillas. Top with Cilantro Crema, Poblano Salsa, or avocado, fresh cilantro and optional pickled onions.

VEGAN RAMEN WITH MISO SHIITAKE BROTH

Vegan Ramen with Miso Shiitake Broth- a delicious healthy ramen recipe with mushrooms, tofu, bok choy, sesame seeds and scallions in the most flavorful broth!

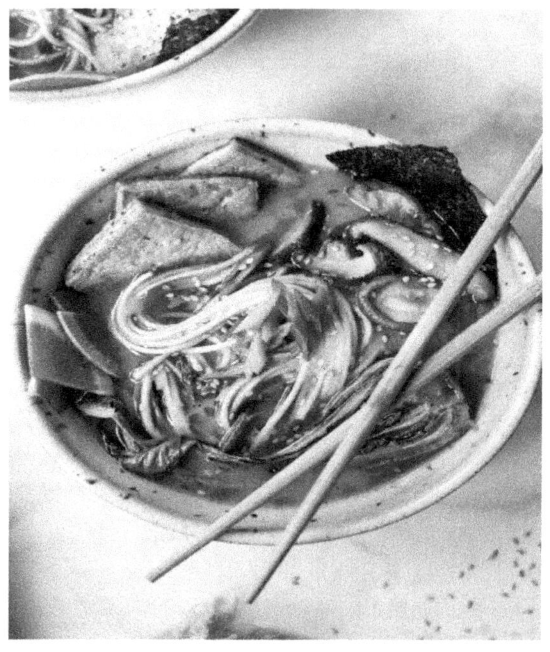

Prep Time	Total Time	Cook Time	Yield
20	1 hour	40	2 serving

Cuisine	Category
Japanese	Vegan, soup, night

Ingredients

Flavorful Vegan Ramen Broth:

- 1 large onion-diced
- 2 smashed garlic cloves
- 1–2 tablespoon olive oil
- 4 cups veggie stock
- 4 cups water
- 1/2 cup dried Shiitake Mushrooms, broken into small pieces
- 1 sheet Kombu seaweed- optional, but good!
- 1/8 cup mirin (Japanese cooking wine)
- 1–2 tablespoons white miso paste
- Pepper to taste
- for spicy, add sriracha to taste, or hot chili oil

Ramen:

- 6– 8 ounces Ramen Noodles
- 8 ounces Cubed Crispy Tofu
- Optional veggies: Steamed or sauteed bok choy, fresh spinach, shredded carrots or cabbage, roasted winter squash, roasted cauliflower, roasted carrots, roasted sweet potato, sauteed mushrooms, smoked mushrooms, baby corn, Bamboo shoots, Enoki mushrooms, Kimchi, Soft boiled eggs (obviously not vegan) daikon radish, pickled radish, fresh herbs.
- Garnishes: scallions, Furikake or toasted sesame seeds, sriracha and sesame oil

Instructions

If adding roasted veggies, do this first. Toss bite-sized pieces, with a little olive oil, salt and pepper and place on a parchment-lined sheet pan and roast in a 400F oven until fork tender.

Make the BROTH: Over medium-high heat, saute the onion in 1 tablespoon oil until tender about 3 minutes. Turn heat to medium, add the smashed garlic cloves and continue cooking the onions until they are deeply golden brown. Add the veggie stock, water, dried shiitakes, a sheet of kombu (rinsed) and mirin. Bring to a Simmer.

Simmer for 25-30 minutes uncovered on med heat, then remove the Kombu. Add the miso, and pepper to taste. Adjust salt to your liking (feel free to add salt, soy or more miso). Keep warm. FYI: If this reduces too much it may become salty…. simply add a little water to taste.

While the broth is simmering, cook the ramen noodles in a pot of boiling water, according to directions. Drain. Toss with sesame oil to keep separated.

Prep other veggies and other toppings. Feel free to steam bok choy or fresh spinach, or saute them until just tender. If using mushrooms, saute in a little oil until tender (or smoke! see post) seasoning with salt and pepper. Use a combo of fresh and cooked veggies for the best texture. Make the crispy tofu!

Assemble Ramen Bowls: Fill bowls with cooked noodles, crispy tofu and any other veggies you want. Pour the flavorful Shiitake broth over top. Garnish with a little drizzle of sesame oil and sriracha. Top with scallions and sesame seeds.

Serve immediately.

SIMPLE BAKED SHEET-PAN RATATOUILLE

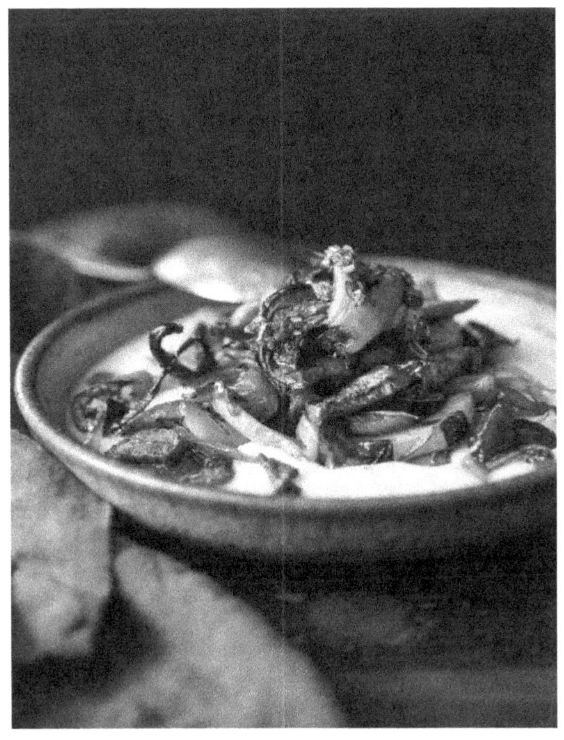

Prep Time:	Total Time	Cook Time	Yield
15	1 hour 15 mins	60	4-6 serving

Category	Cuisine:
Vegan, main, dinner	French

Description

Baked Sheet-Pan Ratatouille is easy, healthy and vegan! Bake a big batch on Sunday then serve it during the busy workweek over pasta, polenta or even toast!

Method: Baked

Ingredients

- 3 Japanese eggplant or one large eggplant
- 1 red or yellow bell pepper
- 2 medium tomatoes
- 2 zucchini or summer squash
- 1 onion
- 8–14 garlic cloves, whole, peeled
- 2–3 tablespoon fresh herbs – thyme or rosemary or combination of both
- olive oil for drizzling
- salt and pepper to taste
- splash balsamic vinegar

Optional Garnishes: Italian parsley or fresh basil ribbons, capers, chili flakes, olive oil

Serve with pasta, soft polenta, whole grains, or feel free to add beans, sausage, chicken.

Easy Creamy Polenta

- 1 cup corn meal
- 4 ½ cups water or stock
- 1 tablespoon olive oil or butter
- ½ cup grated cheese (cheddar, Parmesan, mozzarella, goat cheese)
- salt and pepper to taste

Instructions

Preheat oven to 400 F and place a piece of parchment on 1-2 large sheet pans (I use two).

Using a vegetable peeler, peel eggplant if you want – or just remove some of the skin in long strips. Or if you prefer, leave the skin on. Cut into 1/2 inch thick bite-sized pieces. Slice the bell pepper into ½ inch wide strips. Cut the tomatoes into 3/4 inch wedges. Slice the zucchini the long way and then slice into ½ inch thick half-moons. Slice the onion into ¼-½ inch thick half-moons.

Spread out the veggies on the sheet pan in a single layer (this is why you most likely need two sheet pans). Add whole garlic cloves (peeled) and herbs.

Drizzle with olive oil and toss, using enough oil to coat. Sprinkle with a generous amount of salt and pepper. Toss well.

Roast in the hot oven for 20 minutes, mix the veggies, and roast 20 more minutes, mix again. Turn heat down to 300 and roast 10-20 more minutes, or until tender and edges begin to caramelize.

Taste, adjust salt, and drizzle with a little splash of balsamic vinegar.

Use immediately or cool and refrigerate (or freeze) until ready to use.

SPICY MEXICAN OAXACAN BOWL

Vegan Mexican-style, Oaxacan Bowl with roasted chipotle sweet potatoes and sweet peppers over a bed of warm seasoned black beans. Topped with a crunchy cabbage slaw, avocado and toasted Chipotle Maple Pecans.

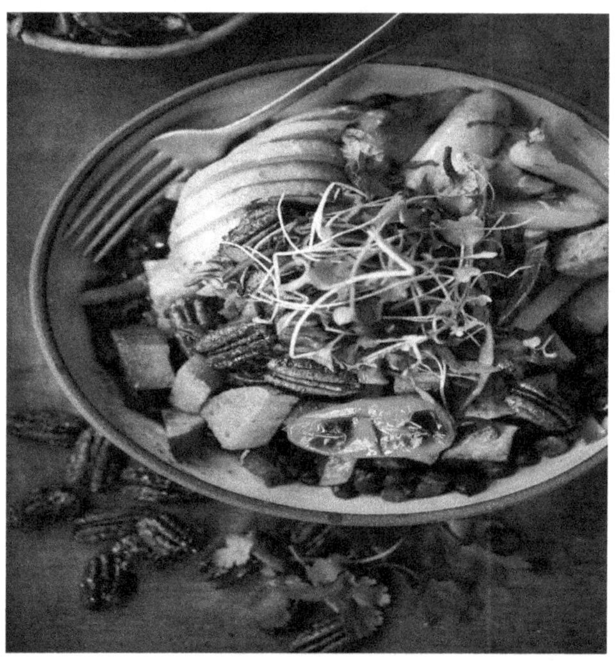

Prep Time	Total Time	Cook Time	Yield
15	40 mins	25	2 servings

Cuisine	Category
Mexican Bowl:	Vegan, main, dinner

Description

Mexican Style Oaxacan Bowl with chipotle sweet potatoes, roasted sweet peppers, seasoned black beans, topped with a cabbage slaw (or Everyday Kale Salad) and toasted chipotle pecans.Vegan and Grain-Free.

Method: Baked

Ingredients

Spice Rub

- 2 teaspoons cumin
- 1 teaspoon ground chipotle (or swap out a mix of smoked paprika and chili powder)
- ½ teaspoon kosher salt

Sheet Pan Ingredients

- ½ a red onion, cut in ½ inch wedges
- 1 medium yam or sweet potato- diced into ¾ inch cubes (leave skin on)
- 8 baby bell peppers, cut in half (or 1 regular red or yellow bell pepper, cut into strips)
- ½ cup pecans
- 2 teaspoons maple syrup
- 15-16 ounce can Seasoned Black Beans (Cuban style or Mexican style) or use regular black beans (see notes)
- Garnish: Avocado, cilantro, scallions, Cabbage Slaw, Mexican Secret Sauce or Vegan Avocado Sauce

Quick Cabbage Slaw

- ¼ of a a red cabbage, shredded
- 1 tablespoon olive oil
- ¼ cup chopped cilantro or scallions or both
- 1 teaspoon coriander
- 1/8 teaspoon kosher salt
- 1 tablespoon lime juice

Instructions

Preheat oven to 400F

Mix cumin, chipotle and salt together in a small bowl.

Place onion, sweet potato and peppers on a parchment lined sheet pan. Drizzle onion and potato with a little olive oil and sprinkle generously with spice mix, tossing to coat all sides well. Use about ½ or ⅔ of the spice.

Place in the oven for 20-30 minutes, tossing halfway through.

On another smaller parchment-lined pan, toss the pecans with 2 teaspoons maple syrup and 1 teaspoon of the spice mix. Place in the oven (on a lower rack) for 7-10 minutes, or until lightly browned. When you pull it out, give nuts a quick toss to loosen them up and "fluffen" them, so when they cool, they are easy to remove.

Heat the seasoned beans in a small pot on the stove (see notes) and make the slaw. Finely chop or shred the cabbage and place in a medium bowl with the rest of the ingredients, toss. Taste, adjust lime and salt.

Slice the avocado.

When the veggies are fork tender, assemble the bowls. Divide the beans among 2-3 bowls. Divide all the veggies, placing them over the beans, and top with slaw and add the avocado.

Serve with the Chipotle Mayo (vegan-adaptable) or Vegan Avocado sauce if you like, or sour cream and hot sauce– it's fine without though too.

PERUVIAN BURRITOS WITH AJI VERDE SAUCE (VEGAN!)

These vegan Peruvian Burritos are filled with roasted sweet potato, fresh corn, peppers, quinoa, whipped black beans, and drizzled with Spicy Peruvian Green Sauce.

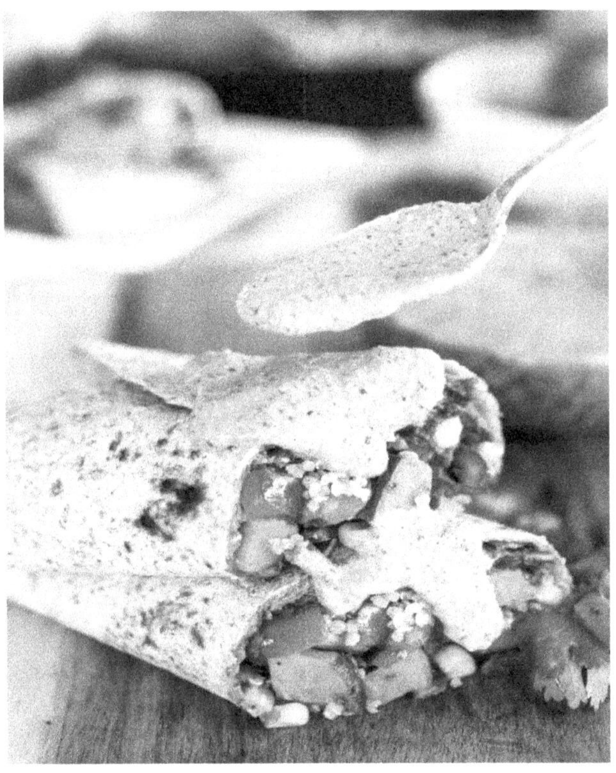

Prep Time	Total Time	Cook Time	Yield
30	1 hour	30	4 serving

Cuisine	Category
Peruvian Diet	Vegan, dinner

Description

Peruvian Burritos with Aji Verde Sauce filled with roasted sweet potato, fresh corn, peppers, quinoa and creamy black beans, then drizzled with spicy Peruvian Green Sauce. A flavor bomb! Vegan and Delicious!

Method: Stove Top and Oven

Ingredients

- 1 small-medium yam or sweet potato, diced (about 1–2 cups)
- olive oil
- salt and pepper to taste
- 3/4 cup dry quinoa (or sub rice)
- 1 1/2 cups water
- 1 tablespoon olive oil
- 1/2 onion, diced
- 4 cloves garlic, rough chopped
- 1 ear of corn, (1 cup corn kernels, or sub 1 cup frozen corn, or 1 cup diced zucchini)
- 1 red bell pepper, diced
- 1 poblano chili
- 1/2 teaspoon salt
- 1 teaspoon cumin
- 1 teaspoon coriander
- 1/2 teaspoon dried oregano
- 1 can refried black beans (or see notes)
- 1 tablespoon oil
- 1 /4 teaspoon salt
- 1/2 teaspoon chili powder
- 1/2 teaspoon cumin

Vegan Aji Verde Sauce:

- 1/3 cup raw cashews

- 1/3 cup water
- 2 garlic cloves
- 1/2 –1 jalapeno (or 1/2 a serrano chili)
- 1/2 teaspoon salt
- 1 1/2 cups cilantro, small stems ok
- 1–2 tablespoon lime juice
- 4 extra-large tortillas (14-16 inches)

Instructions

Preheat oven to 425F and gather ingredients & cut veggies.

Bake Sweet Potatoes: Dice the sweet potatoes into 1/2 inch cubes and place on a parchment-lined sheet pan. Toss with a little olive oil, and a generous five-finger pinch of salt and pepper. Spread out and bake in the middle of the oven until crispy and tender, 20-25 minutes.

Cook Quinoa: At the same time, bring quinoa, water, and pinch of salt to boil in a medium pot. Once boiling, cover, turn heat to low and cook until all the water is gone about 15 minutes. Turn heat off and leave covered. Fluff before serving.

Saute Filling: Also at the same time, in a large skillet, heat oil over medium-high heat. Saute onions 2-3 minutes until they just begin to soften. Add garlic, corn and peppers and lower heat to med, sauteeing until tender, about 10 minutes. Season with the salt, cumin, coriander and oregano. Set aside. When the sweet potatoes are tender, add them to these veggies.

Blend the Peruvian Green Sauce (AJI VERDE SAUCE): While the veggies are sauteeing, blend the Aji Verde ingredients together using a blender. Start with cashews and water, blending till smooth and creamy, scraping down the sides. Add remaining garlic, chili, salt, cilantro and lime juice. Blend until relatively smooth. Scrape it into a small bowl.

Whip The Black Beans: Place 1 can refried black beans into a medium pot, breaking them up with a fork. Add 1/4 cup water (or more) to loosen. Gently warm over medium-low heat, whipping with a fork until they are smooth and creamy. Add a drizzle of olive oil, salt and spices. If you don't care about it being "vegan" stir in grated melty cheese or a dollop of sour cream for extra richness. Whip with fork until creamy and flavorful. You want these to be slightly salty. Cover and turn heat off.

Assemble Burritos: Heat tortillas up until soft and pliable (over a gas flame, or in the oven on the rack). Spread with whipped black beans "the glue", a few tablespoons quinoa, 1/2 cup veggies and 2-3 tablespoon of Peruvian Green Sauce. Roll up, tucking the ends in as best you can. Enjoy!

Peruvian Burrito Bowls: Spoon some warm whipped black beans into the bottom of a bowl. Top with some quinoa, vegges and AJI VERDE Sauce. Garnish with avocado slices, diced tomatoes, cilantro, pumpkin seeds, sunflower sprouts. If making bowls instead of burritos, I would double the beans for 4-6 people.

VEGETARIAN BIRYANI

Quick and easy vegetarian recipe for Biryani! A fragrant Indian rice and chickpea dish infused with Indian spices – vegan adaptable and gluten-free. A quick and easy weeknight meal.

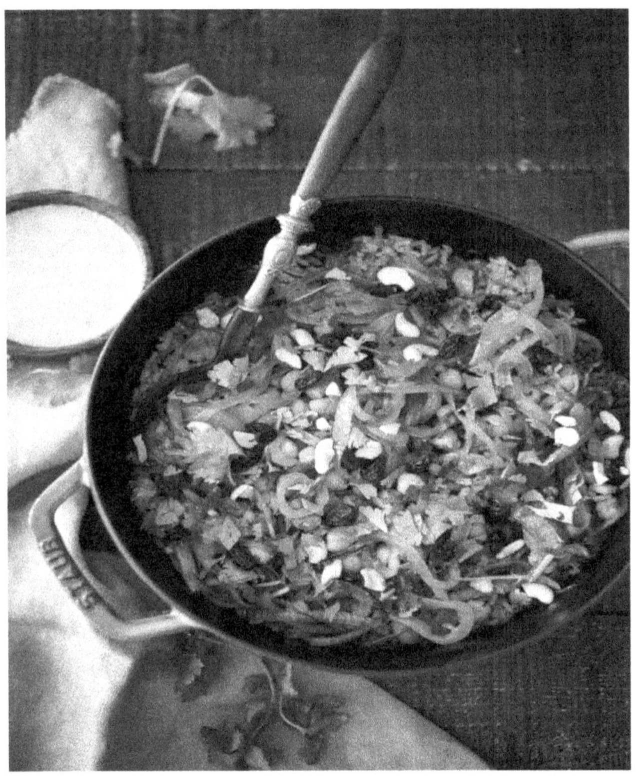

Prep Time	Cook Time	Total Time	Yield
15	30	45 minutes	6 servings

Cuisine	Category

Mexican Bowl   Vegan, Night

Description

Quick and Easy Vegetarian Biryani! A fragrant Indian rice dish infused with Indian spices – vegan adaptable and gluten-free. A quick and easy weeknight meal. Serve it with Cilantro Mint Chutney.

Method: Stove-Top Main

- 2 cups white basmati rice (see notes for brown basmati)
- 2 tablespoons olive oil (or sub ghee or coconut oil)
- 1 large onion, thinly sliced
- 1 red bell pepper, thinly sliced
- 1 cup diced carrot (or use match sticks)
- 4 garlic cloves, rough chopped
- 2 teaspoons fresh ginger, grated or use ginger paste
- 1 tablespoon cumin (or whole seeds)
- 1 tablespoon coriander (or whole seeds, cracked open)
- 1 teaspoon chili powder
- 1 teaspoon cinnamon (or one cinnamon stick)
- 1/2 teaspoon cardamom (or 3 crushed cardamom pods)
- 1/2 teaspoon ground turmeric
- 2 bay leaves
- 1 star anise pod (optional)
- 4 cups veggie stock (or chicken stock)
- 3/4 teaspoon salt, more to taste
- 1 can chickpeas, drained, rinsed
- 1/2 cup raisins

Garnish: 1/4 cup cashews and chopped parsley or cilantro

Instructions

Soak rice in a bowl of hot water while you prep ingredients.

In a large skillet, or shallow Dutch oven, heat oil over medium-high heat. Add the onion and sauté, stirring often, until tender and golden, 5 minutes. Turn heat to medium, add the veggies, garlic and ginger, and saute 4-5 minutes. Remove one cup of the mixture and set aside.

Add spices and bay leaf, and stir one minute, toasting the spices. Drain the rice and add it along with veggie stock and salt.

Top with chickpeas, raisins and the cup of veggies you set aside. Bring to a simmer over high heat, then lower heat to low. Cover the pot with a thin dish towel, then place the lid over the top of the towel, and bring the four corners of the towel up and over the lid. This will tighten the seal and keep the steam in, allowing the rice to cook more quickly and evenly.

Simmer on low 20-30 minutes or until the rice has soaked up the liquid. See notes.

While it is simmering make the Cilantro Mint Chutney

Uncover the Vegetarian Biryani and fluff up with a fork. Top with the toasted cashew and cilantro. Serve with optional Chutney.

FRANKIES

Flavorful Frankie Recipe (an Indian Burrito!) with curry mashed potatoes, chickpeas, cauliflower, spinach, pickled onions and amazing Cilantro Mint Chutney! Vegan and Gluten-free adaptable.

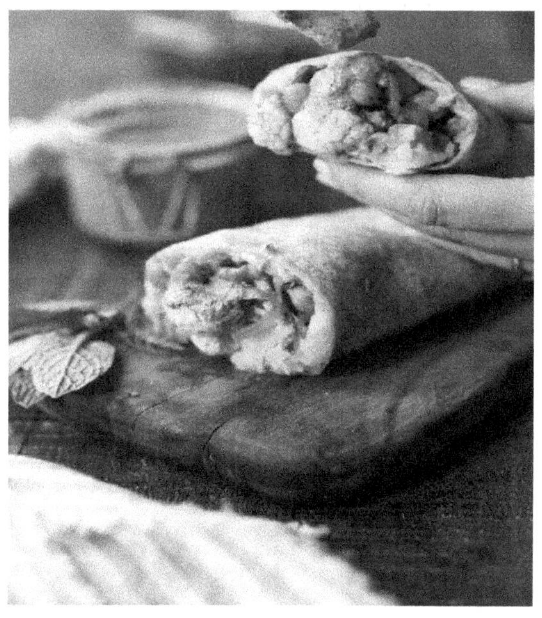

Prep Time	**Cook Time**	**Total Time**	**Yield**
30	30	1 hour	4 servings

Cuisine	**Category**
Mexican Bowl	Vegan,main, dinner

Description

A delicious recipe for Frankies- India's street food, also called a Mumbai Burrito or Bombay Burritos. Filled with curried potatoes, roasted cauliflower and chickpeas, spinach, cilantro mint chutney and pickled onions. Vegan! GF adaptable.

Method: Roasted

Ingredients

Curry Mashed Potatoes (The "Spread")

- 16 ounces baby potatoes – quartered
- 1 tablespoon ghee, olive oil or coconut oil, more to taste
- ¾ teaspoon kosher salt
- 2–3 teaspoons yellow curry powder (see notes)
- 1 teaspoon granulated onion or granulated garlic powder (you could also incorporate sautéed onion and garlic into the potatoes for more flavor)

Roasted Cauliflower & Chickpea (Filling):

- 1 head cauliflower- cut into small florets
- 1 can chickpeas, rinsed and drained well
- 1–2 tablespoons olive oil
- 1 ½ teaspoons kosher salt
- 1 tablespoon coriander
- 1 tablespoon cumin

Generous pinch chili flakes

- 1 teaspoon whole fennel seed (optional, or use cumin seed or coriander seed)
- 1 teaspoon whole coriander seed (optional)

Burrito Fixin's:

- 4 x extra-large, whole wheat tortillas – or feel free to use GF wraps or tortillas, or GF bowls using the mashed potatoes and extra spinach and the base.
- 2 handfuls baby spinach
- Few tablespoons Cilantro Mint Chutney (imperative!!!)
- Few tablespoons Quick Pickled Onions

Instructions

Preheat oven to 425F

Start Potatoes: Cut potatoes and place them in a medium pot, covered with water and simmer until very tender, about 15-20 minutes. At the same time…

Roast Veggies: Cut the cauliflower into small florets and place them on a parchment-lined sheet pan (to one side). Add the drained chickpeas to the other side. Drizzle both with olive oil. Sprinkle cauliflower and chickpeas with the spices and salt, tossing to coat well. Place in the oven and roast for 20-25 minutes tossing halfway through) or until cauliflower is tender.

Sauce: Make the flavorful Cilantro Mint Chutney and quick pickled red onions and place both in jars (of course, you could make these both ahead). They take about 5-10 minutes each. Please don't leave out the mint chutney- it's imperative!!!

Curried Potatoes: Once the potatoes are very tender, drain but save about 1 cup of the hot water. Place the potatoes back in the pot and mash with some of the hot water (start with ¼-½ cup) salt, spices and ghee (or oil) and mash the potatoes to combine until smooth. You want a fairly loose, spreadable mash so add more hot water if necessary. Scrape down the sides. Stir well. Taste. You want this to taste flavorful and slightly salty as the tortilla will mute some of the salt and flavor. Feel free to add more ghee or oil as you please for extra richness. Cover and keep warm.

When the roasted veggies are done, ASSEMBLE: Warm the tortillas either in the oven, over a gas flame or over a grill, until soft and pliable. Spread generously with the curried potatoes, then top with chickpeas, cauliflower making sure to get some of the whole spices that will have dropped to the bottom of the pan. Add a handful of spinach leaves, a few teaspoons of cilantro mint chutney and some pickled onions and roll up like a burrito. Keep warm in the oven until ready to serve, or serve immediately! You can also refrigerate and reheat for meals on the go.

DATE NIGHT VEGAN ALFREDO

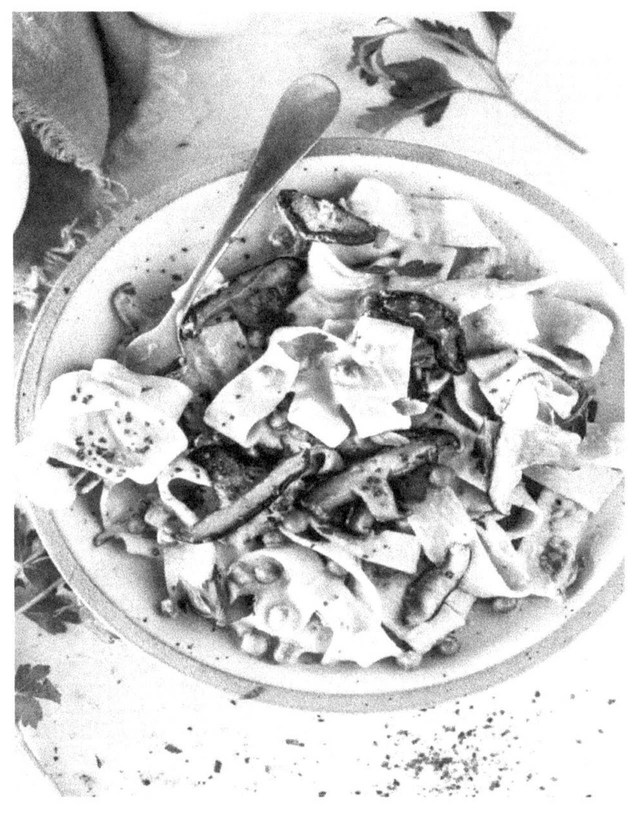

Prep Time	Cook Time:	Total Time	Yield
10	20	30 mins	2 servings

Cuisine	Category
Italian	Vegan, pasta

Description

Date night Vegan Alfredo for two, tossed in a delicious cashew (or hemp) cream, with sauteed mushrooms, Meyer lemon zest and a secret ingredient that gives this extra complexity, flavor and depth. Can be made in under 30 minutes!

Method: stove top

Ingredients

Vegan Alfredo Sauce:

- 1–2 tablespoons olive oil
- 1/2 white onion
- 4 fat garlic cloves
- 1/2 cup raw cashews, soaked (or hemp seeds) see notes
- 1 cup veggie broth (or 1 cup water and boulllion)
- 2 tablespoons nutritional yeast
- 1/2 teaspoon white miso paste
- 1/2 teaspoon salt
- 1/8 teaspoon nutmeg
- 5 ounces dry pasta, cooked to package directions
- 1 cup fresh peas (or frozen, or sub snow peas or steamed broccoli)
- 8 ounces mushrooms, sauteed, or try smoked mushrooms!

Garnish: pepper, chili flakes, lemon zest (Meyer lemons are especially nice), Italian parsley.

Instructions

Cook Pasta: Set salted water to boil in a large pot and cook pasta according to directions. If using fresh or frozen peas, feel free to add to the pasta water, during the last minute of cooking.

Make Alfredo Sauce: Heat oil over med low heat, and saute onion and garlic until tender and golden. Place it in a blender along with cashews, veggie broth, nutritional yeast, miso, salt, nutmeg. Blend until creamy and smooth.

Saute or smoke the mushrooms. If sauteeing, heat olive oil in a skillet over medium heat. Add mushrooms and saute 6-7 minutes, until golden and tender, seasoniong with salt.

Combine: Drain the pasta, add to a large pan along with the alfredo sauce, toss, and gently warm over low heat. Add the mushrooms and toss to coat (leaving a few for the top for garnish if you like).

Divide among two bowls.

Garnish with lemon zest, pepper, chili flakes and chopped parsley.

JALAPEÑO BROCCOLI "CHEDDAR" SOUP (VEGAN)

Jalapeño Broccoli "Cheddar" Soup (vegan) – a fast and easy weeknight meal that is loaded up with lots of healthy broccoli! This delicious soup is vegan, keto and gluten-free- and can be made in 30 minutes!

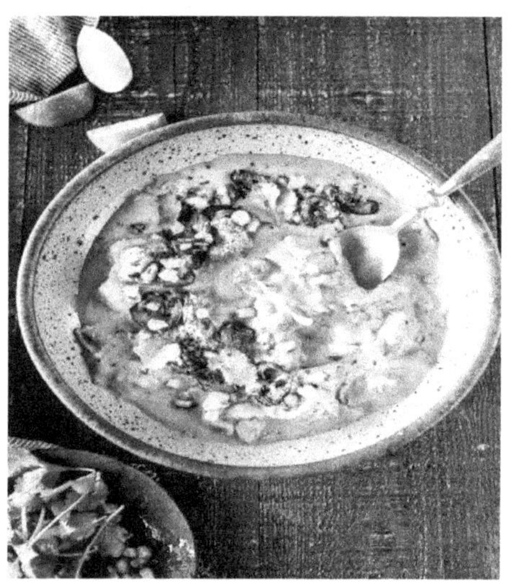

Prep Time	Cook Time	Total Time	Yield
18	20	38 mins	5 servings

Cuisine	Category
Northwest	Vegan, main, dinner, main

Description

Vegan Broccoli "Cheddar" Soup with Jalapeño – a fast and easy weeknight recipe that is healthy, vegan and keto!

Method: Stovetop

Ingredients

- 2 tablespoons olive oil
- 1 large onion, diced
- 4–6 fat garlic cloves, rough chopped
- 1–2 poblano peppers, diced (I like 2)
- 1 jalapeno, diced fine (use 1/2 for less spice- see notes)
- 7 cups broccoli, cut into bite-sized florets (about 1 – 1 ¼ pound, stems ok if cut thinly)
- 4 cups veggie or chicken broth (or 4 cups water + 1 tablespoon "Better than Bouillon" Vegetable Base)
- 1 cup water
- 1 bay leaf (optional, remove before blending)
- 1 teaspoon salt
- 1 teaspoon coriander
- 1 teaspoon oregano
- ½ teaspoon pepper
- 3/4 cup raw cashews (soaked or simmered, see notes) or hemp hearts
- 2–3 tablespoons nutritional yeast (see notes)
- 1–2 large handful baby spinach (for vibrant color)
- **Optional Finishing oil:**
- 2 tablespoons olive oil
- 1 jalapeno sliced
- 1 teaspoon cumin seeds
- pinch chili flakes (optional)
- 1/4 cup corn kernals, frozen is ok (optional)
- 1/4 cup pumpkin seeds (optional)

Optional Garnish:

cilantro or scallions, lime

Instructions

Heat oil in a big pot over medium heat, and add the onion, garlic, poblanos and jalapeno, stirring occasionally, letting the onions get golden, about 5 minutes.

Add the broccoli, broth, water, bay leaf, coriander, oregano, salt, and pepper. The liquid should just cover the veggies. Cover, bring to a boil, turn heat down and simmer gently until broccoli is tender, about 10-12, minutes. Turn heat off and remove bay leaf.

BLEND: Place roughly 1 cup of the broccoli and 1 cup of broth into a blender. Let cool 5 minutes. Add the cashews and 2 tablespoons nutritional yeast.

Cover tightly with blender lid and kitchen towel, holding it down firmly, when you start the motor (on the lowest setting, working up gradually) to prevent a blender "explosion". Blend until silky smooth.

Add one more cup broccoli and one more cup broth. Blend again until silky smooth.

To the blender, add 1-2 big handfuls of fresh baby spinach for that extra vibrant "green" color, and blend until fully incorporated and smooth.

Pour this back in the broccoli soup pot, mix and heat gently over low heat, careful not to boil or simmer too long, or you will lose the lovely vibrant green color.

Taste for salt, heat, and acid. Add a little squeeze of lime if you like, or extra chili flakes or more pepper. For extra "cheesy" flavor add another tablespoon of nutritional yeast.

Make the finishing oil: Heat 2-3 tablespoons olive oil in a small skillet over medium heat. Add sliced jalapeno, 1 teaspoon cumin seeds, chili flakes, and optional corn kernals or pumkin seeds. Heat until cumin is fragrant, about 1 minute. Serve the soup in bowls and spoon a little finishing oil over the soup (when serving) in a crescent shape.

Garnish with fresh cilantro or scallions or a wedge of lime.

GREEK GODDESS BOWL

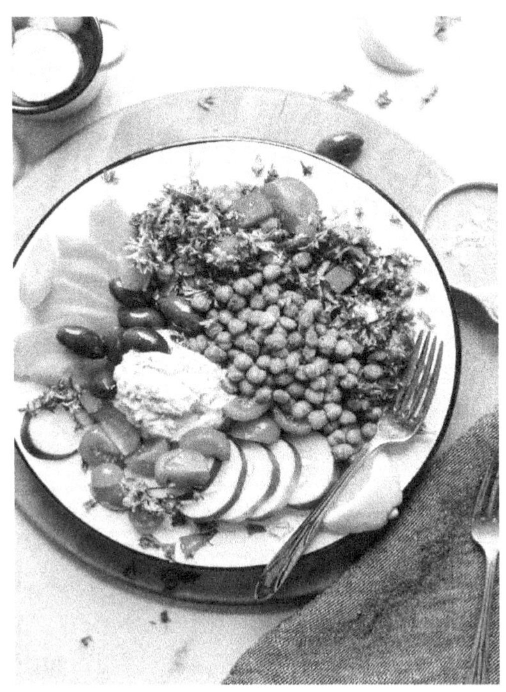

Prep Time	Cook Time	Total Time
7 minutes	23 minutes	30 minutes

Ingredients

Chickpeas

- 1 15-ounce can chickpeas (rinsed, drained and dried well on a towel)
- 1 Tbsp. oil (coconut or avocado are best // omit if avoiding oil)
- 1 Tbsp. shawarma spice blend (or similar spices you have on hand)
- 1 Tbsp. maple syrup or coconut sugar (if avoiding sugar, omit) shawarma spice blend

- 1/4 tsp sea salt

Bowl

- 3/4 cup vegan tzatziki
- 1 batch red pepper hemp tabbouleh(or sub chopped parsley)
- 1/2 cup green or Kalamata olives (pitted and halved/chopped)
- 1/2 cup cherry tomatoes (halved)
- 1 medium cucumber (thinly sliced)
- 1 medium carrot (optional // sliced thinly on a diagonal into "chips")

Instructions

- Preheat oven to 375 degrees F (190 C) and set out a baking sheet.
- Add washed, dried chickpeas to a mixing bowl along with oil, Shawarma Spice Blend, maple syrup, and salt. Toss to combine.
- Add seasoned chickpeas to the baking sheet. Bake for 20-23 minutes or until the chickpeas are slightly crispy and golden brown. Remove from oven and set aside.
- Assemble bowl by dividing tzatziki, tabbouleh (or parsley), olives, tomatoes, cucumber, and carrots (optional) between two serving bowls. Top with cooked chickpeas and garnish with fresh lemon juice.
- This bowl is delicious as is, but it would also pair well with my 4-ingrident garlic dill sauce or my Tahini dressing
- Best when fresh, but you can store leftovers (separately) up to 3-4 days in the refrigerator. Store leftover chickpeas separately in a sealed container at room temperature up to 3 days or in the freezer up to 1 month.

EASY PEANUT NOODLES

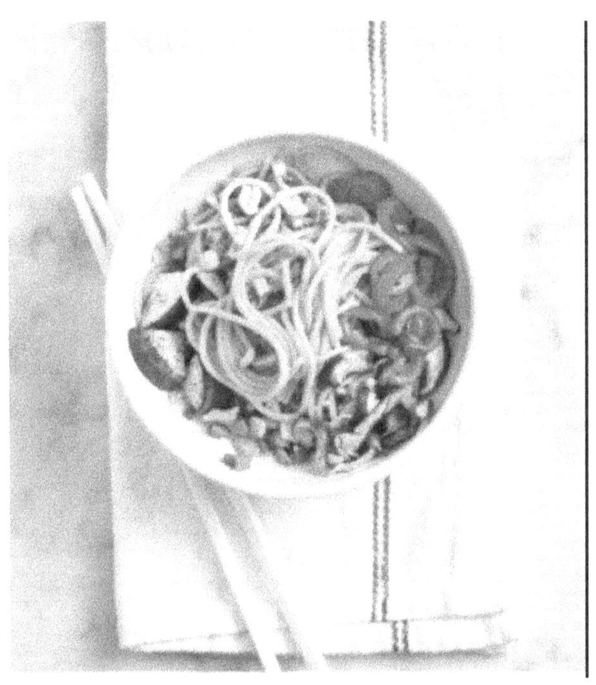

Prep time	Cook time	Total time	Serves:
15 mins	15 mins	30 mins	2 to 3

Ingredients

- 8 ounces soba noodles, pasta, or rice noodles
- Shiitake mushrooms
- Eggplant
- Red peppers
- Chopped scallions
- Sesame seeds
- Peanut Sauce
- Crushed peanuts

Instructions

- Cook your noodles according to the package directions.
- Heat a skillet to medium, add a little oil. Add the mushrooms & eggplant and let cook for a few minutes until the mushrooms and eggplant become soft. Add the red pepper and scallions and cook for a few minutes more. Add a splash of soy sauce and remove the pan from the heat.
- Toss noodles with peanut sauce and add the veggies.
- Top with sesame seeds and crushed peanuts. Serve warm or cold.

HOMEMADE SPAGHETTI O'S (ALLERGY-FREE, GLUTEN-FREE, VEGAN)

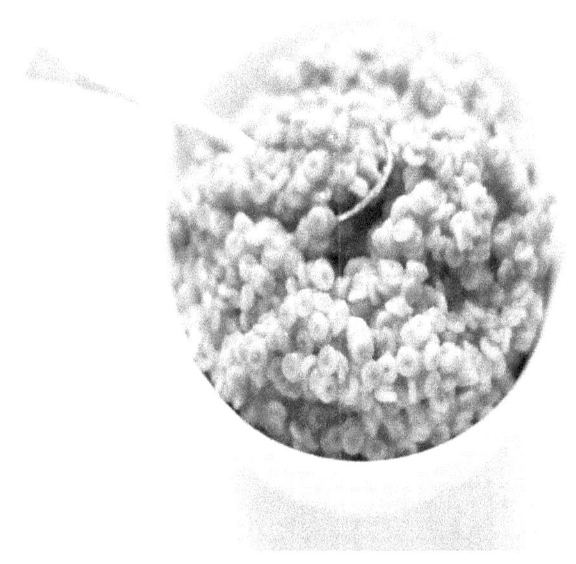

Cook Time	Total Time	Yield	Category
10 mins	10 mins	4-6 1x	Main

Ingredient

- 1 (12oz) Box gluten-free anellini pasta
- 1 (15oz) Can no-salt added tomato sauce
- ⅓ Cup Unsweetened Non-Dairy Milk
- ¼ Cup nutrition yeast
- 2 TB tomato paste
- 1 Tsp onion powder

- ½ Tsp garlic powder
- ½ Tsp paprika

Instructions

- In a large pot, cook pasta according to box directions, drain, and add back into pot.
- Now add all other ingredients to the pot, with heat turned to low and mix well to combine.
- Serve warm or cold!

BURRITO STUFFED PEPPERS

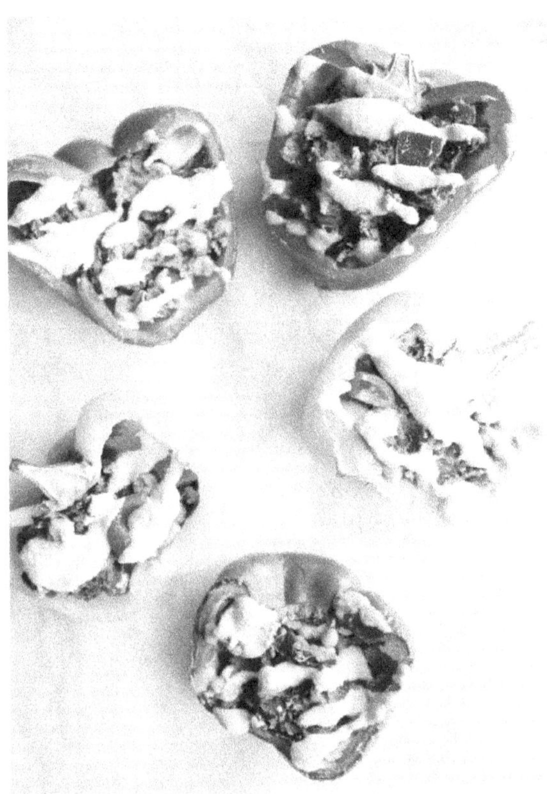

Prep Time	Cook Time	Total Time	Yield
8 minutes	25 minutes	33 minutes	3

Ingredients

- 3 bell peppers
- 1 tbsp. olive oil
- 2 cloves garlic, minced
- 3 spring onions, sliced
- ½ tsp chili powder
- 1 x 400g tins kidney or black beans, drained and rinsed
- 1 large tomato, diced

- 1 small tin, approx. 150g of sweetcorn, drained and rinsed
- Salt and pepper, to taste

Instructions

- Preheat the oven to 180C / 350F.
- Chop the bell peppers in half and remove the seeds. Add to a roasting tin and drizzle with olive oil. Cook for approximately 15-20 minutes until slightly browned and softened but still firm enough to retain its shape.
- Meanwhile, add the garlic, onion and a small splash of water to a frying pan. Cook on a medium heat for a minute, then add the chili powder and beans. Add some more water (about a tablespoon or two) and cook for a few minutes, until the beans are softened and moist. Partially mash them with a fork or masher so you have a chunky bean paste.
- Stir in the chopped tomato, sweetcorn and salt & pepper.
- Spoon the mixture into the pepper halves and return to the oven for another 5-8 minutes, just too warm through.
- Serve hot with the vegan cashew cheese sauce drizzled on top. Enjoy!

EASY VEGAN CAULIFLOWER FRIED RICE

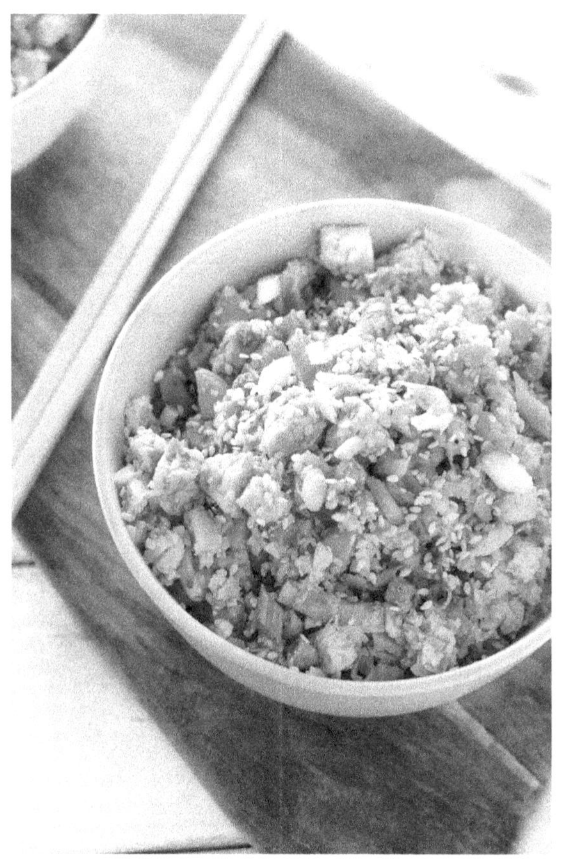

Prep Time	Cook Time	Total Time	Yield
15 Minutes	15 Minutes	30 Minutes	4 Servings

Ingredients

- 1 lb. firm tofu and drained
- 1 medium-sized head of cauliflower
- 2 tablespoons sesame oil, divided
- 1 tablespoon minced ginger

- 3 cloves garlic, minced
- 2 carrots, diced (about 1 cup)
- 1/2 cup peas, thawed if frozen
- 1/4 cup thinly sliced green onions
- 3 tablespoons cashews
- 3 tablespoons soy sauce (or Tamari for gluten-free version)
- sesame seeds, for garnish

Instruction

- Press and drain the tofu [either by wrapping the tofu in paper towels or placing under a heavy object]
- Lightly crumble the tofu in a large bowl and set aside.
- Cut the cauliflower into florets, discarding the tough inner core. Working in batches if needed, pulse the cauliflower in a food processor until it breaks down into rice-sized pieces. You should have 5 to 6 cups of cauliflower "rice."
- Set aside.
- In a large wok, heat the sesame oil over medium heat. Add the ginger and garlic and lightly stir fry for 30 seconds – 1 minute until just golden brown and fragrant. Add in the crumbled tofu and stir-fry for 5 minutes, stirring often, until tofu is golden in color and cooked through.
- Remove tofu from wok and add the remaining 1 tablespoon of sesame oil.
- Add in the carrots and sauté until tender, about 2 minutes. Stir the peas, and cauliflower "rice" into the wok, mixing the ingredients thoroughly.
- Cook, stirring often, until the cauliflower is tender, 5 to 8 minutes. Stir in the cooked tofu, green onions, cashews and soy sauce.
- Garnish with sesame seeds, if desired.

NOODLE-FREE PAD THAI

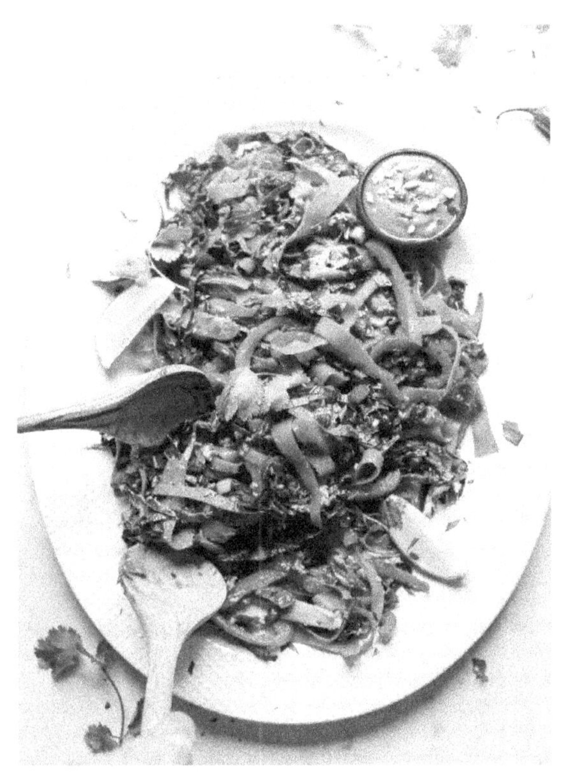

Prep Time	Cook Time	Total Time
15 minutes	15 minutes	30 minutes

Servings	Course	Cuisine	Freezer Friendly	Does it keep
2/4	Entree	Gluten-Free, Thai-Inspired, Vegan	No	2-3 Days

Ingredients

TOFU optional

- 1/2 cup extra-firm tofu (excess liquid pressed out, crumbled with a fork)
- 1 Tbsp. coconut amino (or tamari or soy sauce if not GF)
- 1 tsp chili garlic sauce (or 1/8 tsp red pepper flake as original recipe is written)
- 1/4 tsp ground turmeric (optional)

Sauce

- 2 1/2 Tbsp. nut butter (almond butter, peanut butter, sunflower seed butter, etc.)
- 3 Tbsp. lime juice
- 3 1/2 Tbsp. **coconut amino** (or sub tamari or soy sauce if not GF // plus more to taste)
- 1/2 tsp red pepper flake (or sub 1 tsp chili garlic sauce- Huy Fong Foods brand)
- 1 1/2 Tbsp. maple syrup (12 g coconut sugar // plus more to taste)

Veggies

- 1 Tbsp. sesame oil (sub water or omit if low/no-fat)
- 1 medium serrano pepper (seeds + stem removed, thinly sliced // omit for less heat)
- 1 small bundle green onions (ends removed + thinly sliced)
- 1 1/2 cups thinly sliced red cabbage
- 1 medium red bell pepper (cored and thinly sliced lengthwise)
- 2 Tbsp. coconut amino (or tamari or soy sauce if not gluten free // divided)
- 4-5 large carrots (peeled and rib boned with a vegetable peeler // ~4 cups packed)
- 6 leaves collard greens (large stems removed, stacked + thinly sliced // ~2 cups packed)
- 1/2 tsp freshly grated ginger (*optional* // or 1/4 tsp ground ginger as original recipe is written)

- 1/2 tsp freshly grated turmeric (*optional* // or 1/4 tsp ground turmeric)

Instructions

- If serving with tofu: Add tofu to a small mixing bowl and season with coconut amino, chili garlic sauce (or pepper flake), and turmeric (optional). Stir and set aside.
- Add all sauce ingredients to a small mixing bowl and whisk to combine. Taste and adjust flavor as needed, adding more lime juice for acidity, coconut amino for saltiness, red pepper flake or chili sauce for heat, or maple syrup for sweetness. Set aside.
- Heat a large skillet over medium heat. Once hot, add oil (or water), pepper, onions, cabbage, bell pepper, and half of the coconut amino for veggies (1 Tbsp. as original recipe is written). Cook for 3 minutes, stirring/tossing frequently.
- Add tofu to a corner of the pan and sauté until slightly browned, stirring frequently – about 3-5 minutes.
- Add carrots and collard greens and remaining half of the coconut amino for the veggies (1 Tbsp. as original recipe is written) and stir. Sauté for 2 minutes. Then add Pad Thai sauce and freshly grated ginger and turmeric (optional).
- Sauté over medium heat until warmed through and collards are slightly wilted – about 3 minutes – stirring frequently.
- Taste and adjust flavor of dish as needed, adding more maple syrup for sweetness, red pepper flake or chili garlic for heat, coconut amino for saltiness, or lime juice for acidity.
- Divide between serving plates and enjoy. Serve as is or with peanut sauce, crushed peanuts, cilantro, and lime wedges. Serves 2 as an entrée or 4 as a side.

ROASTED CAULIFLOWER STEAKS

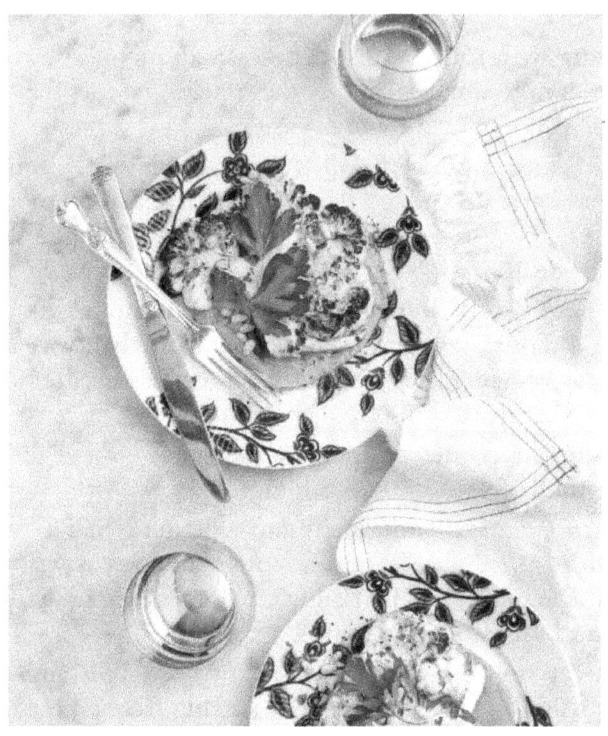

Prep time	Cook time	Total time
15 mins	20 mins	35 mins

Ingredients

- 2 1-inch thick cauliflower "steaks" from 1 medium cauliflower
- 1 tablespoon sunflower oil (or other high-heat oil)
- Sea salt and freshly ground black pepper
- 2 tablespoons chopped parsley
- 2 tablespoons pine nuts, toasted
- 1 tablespoon golden raisins
- ½ teaspoon lemon zest

ROMESCO SAUCE: (THIS MAKES EXTRA)

- 2 roasted red bells peppers, fresh or from a jar
- 2 tablespoons tomato paste
- 3 tablespoons water
- 2 tablespoons red wine vinegar
- ¼ cup cooked chickpeas (or 1 slice ciabatta bread, for thickening)
- ¼ cup toasted hazelnuts
- ¼ cup blanched almonds
- 2 garlic cloves
- 1 teaspoon sweet paprika
- ¼ cup extra-virgin olive oil, more to taste
- Sea salt and freshly ground black pepper

Instructions

- Make the Romesco Sauce: In a blender, combine the red peppers, tomato paste, water, vinegar, chickpeas, hazelnuts, almonds, garlic, paprika, olive oil, and a pinch of salt and pepper. Blend until smooth. Season to taste.

- Preheat the oven to 400°F. Cut two 1-inch thick slices from the cauliflower, keeping the core intact. Heat the oil in a large cast iron pan. Place the cauliflower steaks into the pan and gently press them down. Lightly brush the top of the steaks with a little more oil, and season with salt and pepper. Sear for 2 minutes per side, or until golden brown, then transfer to the oven and roast for 15 minutes or until the cauliflower is tender but firm.

- Spread two plates with romesco sauce and top each with a cauliflower steak. Sprinkle with the chopped parsley, pine nuts, golden raisins, and lemon zest. Season with salt and pepper to taste.

- Store extra romesco sauce in the fridge for up to 4 days. Slather it on sandwiches or use as a veggie dip.

STICKY GINGER SESAME TOFU AND VEGGIES

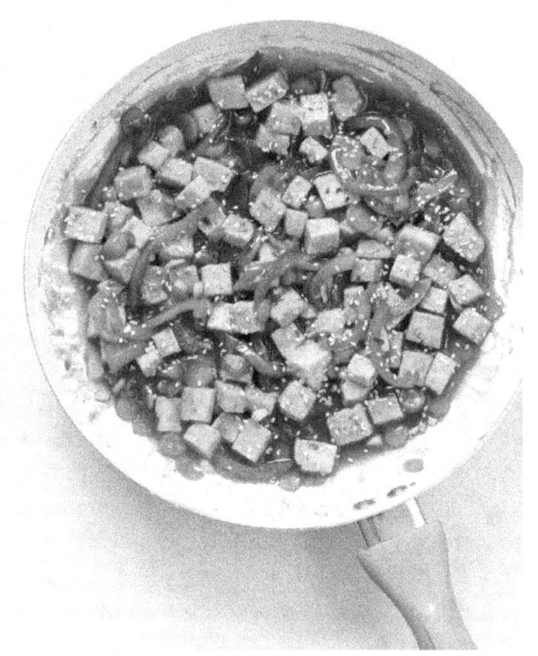

Prep Time	Cook Time	Total Time
10 mins	20 mins	30 mins

Ingredients

Noodles:

- 6 oz (170.1 g) brown rice vermicelli or maifun or rice noodles
- 1 tsp lime juice or lemon

- 1/2 tsp (0.5 tsp) toasted sesame oil
- 1/4 tsp (0.25 tsp) red pepper flakes optional

Sticky Sesame Tofu:

- 1 tsp oil
- 12 to 14 oz (340.2 g) firm tofu
- 2 tsp sesame oil
- 1/2 (0.5) large red bell pepper thinly sliced
- 1/2 (0.5) or 1 large green bell pepper thinly sliced
- 1 hot chile green (Serrano) or red(birds eye)
- 1/2 cup (64 g) sliced carrots
- 1/2 to 1 cup (91 g) other veggies of choice
- 5 cloves of garlic finely chopped
- 1 tbsp minced ginger peel ginger and mince
- 1/3 cup (77.33 ml) soy sauce or tamari
- 1/4 cup (80.5 g) maple syrup
- 2 to 3 tbsp rice vinegar
- 2 to 3 tsp sriracha
- 1 tbsp orange juice optional
- a generous dash of black pepper
- 1/4 tsp (0.25 tsp) salt
- 1 tbsp cornstarch or use arrowroot starch
- 1/4 to 1/2 cup (62.5 ml) water
- cilantro for garnish 1 tbsp toasted sesame seeds

Instructions

- Prepare the vermicelli/rice noodles according to instructions on the package. Rinse in Cold water and transfer to a bowl. Add a dash of lemon or lime juice, pepper flakes and 1/2 tsp sesame oil(optional) and toss. Divide into 2 or 3 serving bowls.
- Wrap the tofu in paper towel and then a kitchen towel. Place a heavy book on it for 5 minutes. unwrap and cube into small cubes. (or press using tofu press and cube)
- Heat 1 tsp oil in a skillet over medium heat. When hot, add the cubed tofu and cook for 5 to 7 minutes until golden on some sides. Transfer to a bowl.
- Add sesame oil, peppers, chile pepper and other veggies if using. Cook for 3 to 4 minutes.

- Add garlic and ginger and cook for 3 minutes. Stir occasionally
- Add the sauce ingredients till salt and mix. Add the crisped tofu and bring the mixture to a good rolling boil. 3 to 4 minutes
- Mix cornstarch with water in a bowl to make a slurry. Add cornstarch slurry and continue to cook until the sauce thickens. Taste adjust heat and sweet. Add some coconut sugar/sweetener or cayenne if needed.
- Divide into the serving bowls.. Garnish with toasted sesame seeds, pepper flakes and cilantro. Add crunchy sides as sliced cucumber, sprouts or carrots.

QUINOA GADO-GADO BOWL (30 MINUTES!)

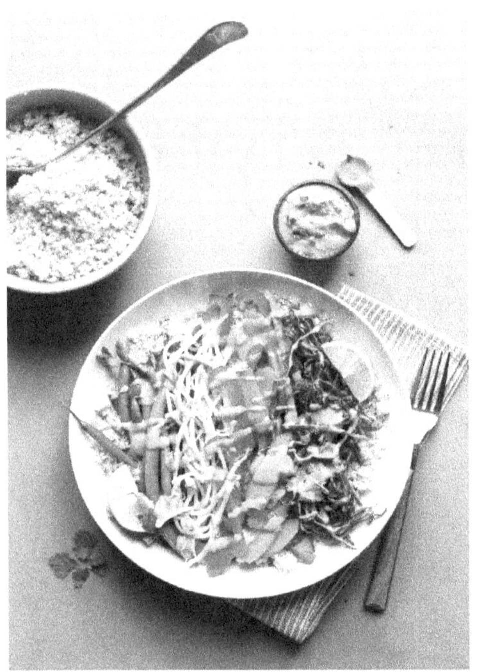

Prep Time	Cook Time	Total Time
7 minutes	23 minutes	30 minutes

Ingredients

Gado-Gado

- 1/2 cup white or red quinoa (well rinsed and drained)
- 1 cup water
- 1 cup greens beans (trimmed)
- 1/2 medium red bell pepper (thinly sliced)
- 3/4 cup mung bean sprouts
- 2/3 cup thinly shredded red cabbage
- 2 whole carrots (thinly sliced with a knife or mandolin)

Spicy Peanut Sauce

- 1/3 cup salted creamy peanut butter (or sub almond butter, cashew butter, or sun butter)
- 1 Tbsp gluten-free tamari (or soy sauce if not GF)
- 2-3 Tbsp maple syrup (to taste)
- 3 Tbsp lime juice
- 1 tsp **chili garlic sauce** (more to taste // 1 Thai red chili, minced // or 1/4 tsp red pepper flake // amounts as original recipe is written)
- 3-4 Tbsp water (to thin)

Instructions

- Heat a small saucepan over medium heat and add rinsed, drained quinoa. "Toast" for 3-4 minutes, stirring frequently, to remove excess liquid and add a nutty flavor to the quinoa. Then add water, stir, and bring to a low boil. Then reduce heat to a simmer, cover, and cook for about 18-20 minutes or until all liquid is absorbed and quinoa is tender. Fluff with a fork, remove lid, and set off heat.

- While quinoa is cooking, steam green beans until just tender. You can do this either in the microwave (covered, in 1-minute increments) or by placing green beans in a steamer basket inside a large saucepan filled with 1 inch of water. Bring the water to a simmer on medium-high heat, cover, and cook until just tender – about 4 minutes.

- Once steamed, add green beans to a bowl of ice water to "shock" them (stop them from cooking). Set aside.

- Make peanut sauce by adding peanut butter, tamari, maple syrup, lime juice, and chili garlic sauce/Thai chili/red pepper flake to a small mixing bowl and whisking to combine. Then add water 1 Tbsp (15 ml) at a time until a semi-thick but pourable sauce is formed.

- Taste and adjust flavor as needed, adding more tamari for saltiness, lime juice for acidity, maple syrup for sweetness, or chili garlic sauce/Thai chili/red pepper flake for heat! You want this to be a balance of tangy, sweet, salty, and spicy, so don't be shy with the seasonings!

- To serve, divide quinoa between 2 serving bowls (as original recipe is written // adjust if altering batch size) and top with green beans, red bell pepper, mung bean sprouts, and carrots. Serve with peanut sauce and any additional toppings (optional), such as cilantro, lime wedges, and red pepper flake.
- Store leftovers separately in the refrigerator up to 4-5 days (peanut sauce keeps for 1+ week). Best when fresh.

SPICY VEGAN ORANGE GROUND CHIK'N BOWLS

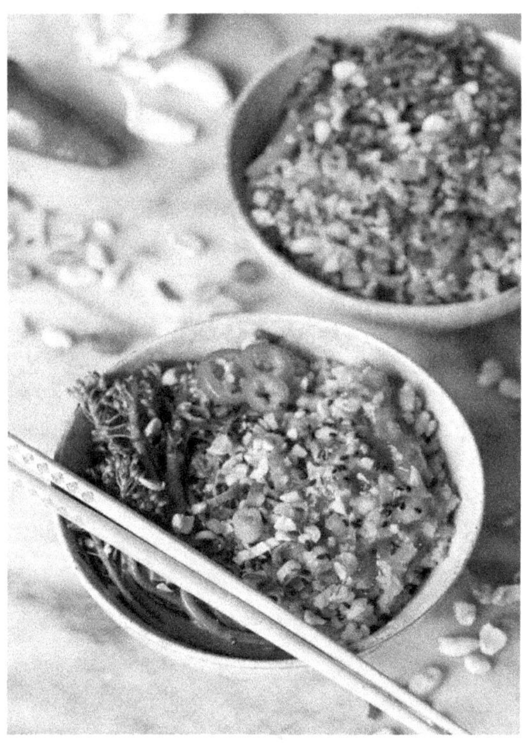

Prep Time	Cook Time	Total Time
15 minutes	20 minutes	35 minutes

Ingredients

Orange chili sauce

- 1 cup water
- 3 tbsp pure maple syrup See Note
- 2 tbsp chili sauce See Note
- 1 tbsp fresh ginger grated

- 1 tbsp Nielsen-Massey Pure Orange Extract See Note
- ½ tsp Nielsen-Massey Pure Lemon Extract
- ¼ cup water plus 1 tbsp corn starch

Chik'n mixture

- 1 tsp sesame oil optional See Note
- 1 small yellow onion finely diced
- 3 garlic cloves minced
- 14 oz chicken flavored seitan ground
- 1 bunch broccolini
- 1 cup uncooked rice cook according to directions on the package
- Sesame seeds optional
- Garnish
- crushed peanuts
- chopped green onion and sesame seeds

Instructions

- Cook the rice.
- Orange Sauce
- Whisk the ¼ cup (60 ml) water and corn starch in a small bowl until the corn starch is fully dissolved.
- In a small saucepan, Whisk the water, maple syrup, chili sauce, ginger, orange extract and lemon extract until combined. Bring to a boil and whisk in the corn starch mixture. Reduce the heat to simmer and cook for 3 to 5 minutes, or until it thickens. Remove from the heat.
- Steam the broccolini for approximately 5 minutes, or until the stalks are fork tender.

Chik'n Seitan

- Grind the seitan in a food processor or with a chef's knife.
- In a large skillet, heat the oil and add the onions when the oil is hot. Cook for approximately 5 minutes, or until they begin to become translucent. Stir often. Add the seitan and garlic and stir to combine, cook for 2 minutes. Add the sauce and stir to coat the seitan. Add the broccolini and sauté for 2 to 4 minutes, or until heated through.
- Build your bowl to suit your style. Garnish with peanuts, green onion, and sesame seeds for extra crunch.

CHIMICHURRI CAULIFLOWER STEAKS

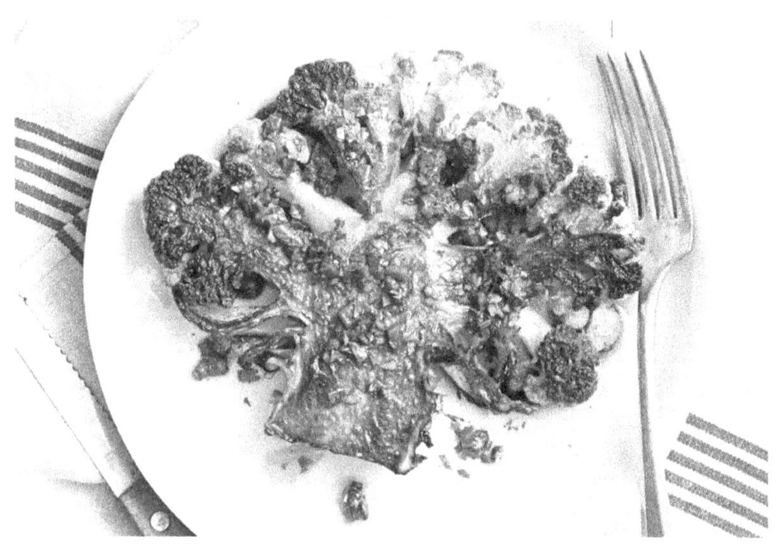

Yields	Prep Time	Total Time
2	0 hours 5 mins	0 hours 20 mins

Ingredients

- 1 Large head cauliflower
- 1 tsp Ground cumin
- 5 tbsp Canola oil
- 1/4 c Loosely packed cilantro, finely chopped
- 1/4 c Loosely packed fresh parsley leaves, finely chopped
- 3 tbsp Red wine vinegar
- 1 Small clove garlic, crushed with press
- 1 Jalapeño Chile, seeded and finely chopped

Instruction

- Trim leaves and any excess stem from cauliflower. Stand cauliflower on stem end and slice off about ¼ inch. Cut 2 slices from center of cauliflower (each about 1 inch thick); reserve rounded wedges for another use.
- Combine cumin and 1 tbsp. canola oil. Brush all over cauliflower slices.
- Sprinkle with ¼ tsp. salt.
- In 12-inch oven-safe skillet, heat 2 tbsp. oil on medium-high until hot.
- Add cauliflower; cook 3 minutes. Turn slices over.
- Place skillet in 425°F oven; roast 15 to 20 minutes or until stem is tender when pierced with tip of paring knife.
- Meanwhile, stir together cilantro, parsley, vinegar, garlic, jalapeño, remaining 2 tbsp. oil, and ⅛ tsp. salt.
- Spoon herb sauce onto finished "steaks."

ZUCCHANOUSH

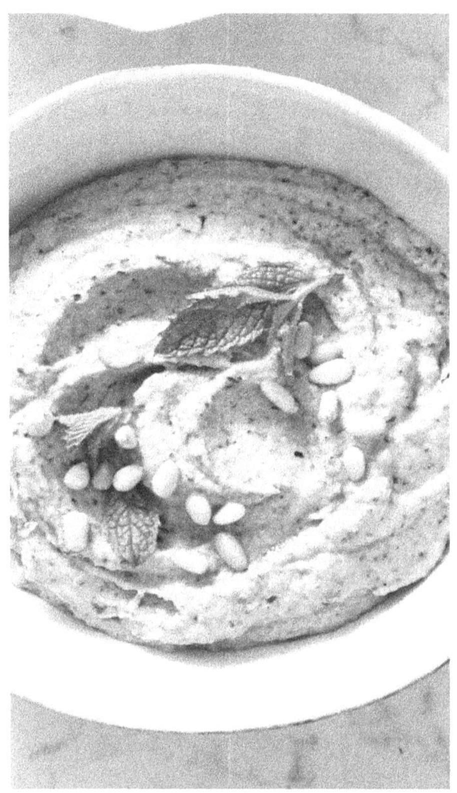

Cal/Serv	Yields	Total Time
125	7 servings	0 hours 15 mins

Ingredients

- 1 lb small zucchini (about 3), quartered lengthwise
- 3 tbsp.olive oil, divided
- Kosher salt and pepper
- 1 clove garlic
- 1/4 c tahini
- 2 tbsp. fresh lemon juice
- 3 tbsp. mint leaves, divided

- 1 tbsp pine nuts, toasted

Instruction

- Heat grill to medium. Toss zucchini with 1 tablespoon oil and 1/2 teaspoon salt and grill until tender and evenly charred, 8 to 10 minutes.
- Transfer zucchini to blender along with garlic, tahini, lemon juice, and 1 tablespoon mint and pulse to combine. With motor running on low speed, drizzle in remaining 2 tablespoons olive oil and puree until mostly smooth, increasing blender speed if necessary.
- Chop remaining mint. Serve zucchini mixture topped with mint and pine nuts.

CREAMY ROASTED SQUASH PUREE

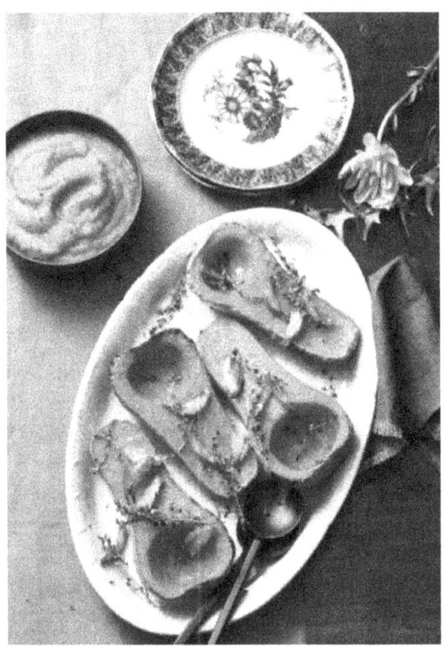

Cal/Serv	Yields	Total Time
215	8	1 hour 30 mins

Ingredients

- 3 tbsp olive oil, divided, plus more for foil
- 3 butternut squash (about 2 pounds each)
- Kosher salt and pepper
- 8 small shallots, quartered
- 12 sprigs fresh thyme, plus more for serving
- 3 tbsp pure maple syrup

Instruction

- Heat oven to 400°F. Line rimmed baking sheet with foil; oil foil.

- Cut butternut squash lengthwise in half and scoop out and discard seeds. Working on prepared baking sheet, coat squash with 2 tablespoons oil and season with 3/4 teaspoon salt and 1/4 teaspoon pepper. Turn squash cut sides down and roast in lower half of oven until flesh is beginning to turn golden brown, 30 to 35 minutes.

- Meanwhile, toss shallots and thyme with remaining tablespoon oil and 1/4 teaspoon each salt and pepper. Turn squash, scatter shallots and thyme on top, then drizzle with maple syrup. Roast until skin is golden brown and crisp, 40 to 50 minutes more.

- Let sit until cool enough to handle. Working in batches, scoop some of the softened squash and shallots from the peels into a food processor and puree until smooth.

CUCUMBER-MELON SOUP

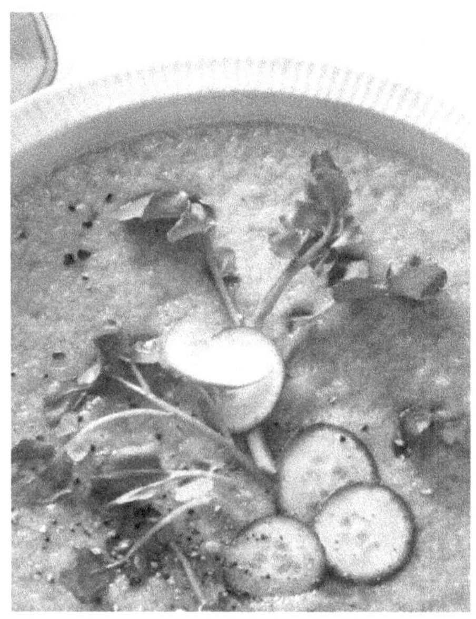

Cal/Serv	Yields	Total Time
75	4 servings	0 hours 45 mins

Ingredients

- 1 lb English cucumbers, cut into pieces, plus more for serving
- 1/2 small honeydew melon, seeded and rind removed (about 1 pound), cut into pieces
- 1/2 c flat-leaf parsley
- 3 tbsp red wine vinegar
- 1 tbsp fresh lime juice
- 2 tsp sugar
- Kosher salt and pepper
- Watercress, for serving

Instruction

- In blender, puree cucumbers, melon, parsley, vinegar, lime juice, sugar, and 1/2 teaspoon salt until smooth.
- Refrigerate at least 1 hour and up to overnight. Serve topped with watercress, sliced cucumber, and cracked pepper.

GRILLED ASPARAGUS AND SHITAKE TACOS

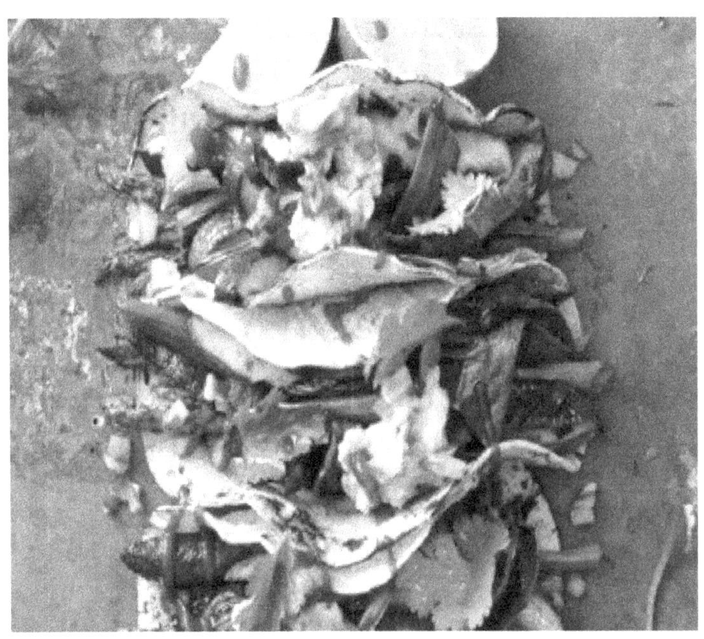

Yields	Prep Time	Total Time
4	0 hours 15 mins	0 hours 20 mins

Ingredients

- 3 tbsp. canola oil
- 4 garlic cloves, crushed with press
- 1 tsp. ground chipotle chile
- 1/2 tsp. Kosher salt
- 8 oz. shiitake mushrooms, stems discarded
- 1 bunch green onions, trimmed
- 8 corn tortillas, warmed
- 1 c. homemade or prepared guacamole
- Lime wedges

- cilantro sprigs
- Hot sauce, for serving

Instruction

- Heat grill on medium. In a large baking dish, combine oil, garlic, chipotle, and salt. Add asparagus, shiitakes, and green onions; toss to coat. Grill asparagus until tender and lightly charred, turning occasionally; 5 to 6 minutes. Grill shiitakes and green onions until lightly charred, turning occasionally; 4 to 5 minutes. Transfer vegetables to cutting board.
- Cut asparagus and green onions into 2" lengths and slice shiitakes. Serve with corn tortillas, guacamole, lime wedges, cilantro, and hot sauce.

BURGERS RECIPE

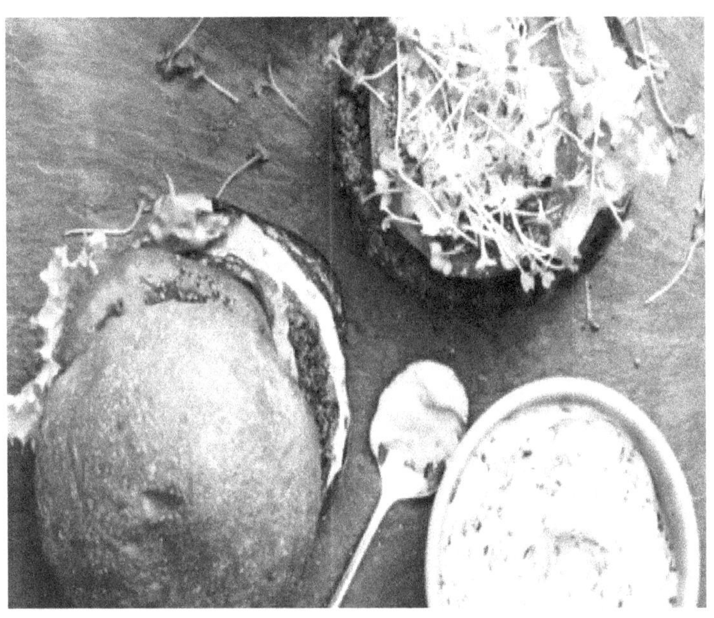

Yields	Prep Time	Total Time
5 servings	0 hours 15 mins	0 hours 45 mins

Ingredients

Burgers

- 4 medium Portobello mushroom caps (about 1 lb.), gills removed, chopped
- 1/2 c. walnuts
- 1 clove garlic
- 2 tbsp. canola oil
- 1/4 c. Chopped red onion
- 3 green onions, chopped
- 2 tsp. rice wine vinegar
- 1 c. cooked quinoa
- 1/2 c. cornstarch

- Whole-grain burger buns
- Sprouts
- Lettuce
- Sliced tomatoes
- 1/2 c. mayonnaise
- 1 tsp. finely chopped fresh rosemary
- 1 tsp. lemon juice
- Kosher salt

Instruction

- **Make the Burgers:** Preheat oven to 375 degrees F. In 3-quart, shallow baking dish, toss mushrooms with walnuts, garlic, 1 tablespoon oil, 3/4 teaspoon salt, and 1/4 teaspoon pepper; spread in even layer. Bake 20 minutes or until mushrooms are tender. Set aside to cool. Turn oven off.
- In food processor, pulse mushroom mixture, red onion, green onions, and vinegar until mostly smooth, scraping side of bowl if necessary. Transfer mixture to a large bowl and stir in quinoa and cornstarch until well-blended. Cover bowl with plastic wrap and refrigerate 2 hours.
- Preheat oven to 375 degrees F. Line baking sheet with foil. Form mixture into 5 patties (about 1/2" thick and 3" wide). In a 12" nonstick skillet, heat remaining 1 tablespoon oil on medium. In 2 batches, cook patties 5 minutes or until well-browned, turning over once. Transfer seared patties to prepared baking sheet. Bake 10 minutes or until hot in centers.
- **Make the Rosemary Mayo:** Meanwhile, combine mayonnaise, rosemary, lemon juice, and a pinch of salt. Keeps up to 5 days, refrigerated.
- Serve burgers on buns with Rosemary Mayo, garnished with sprouts, lettuce, and tomato.

SPICED FRESH TOMATO SOUP WITH SWEET AND HERBY PITAS

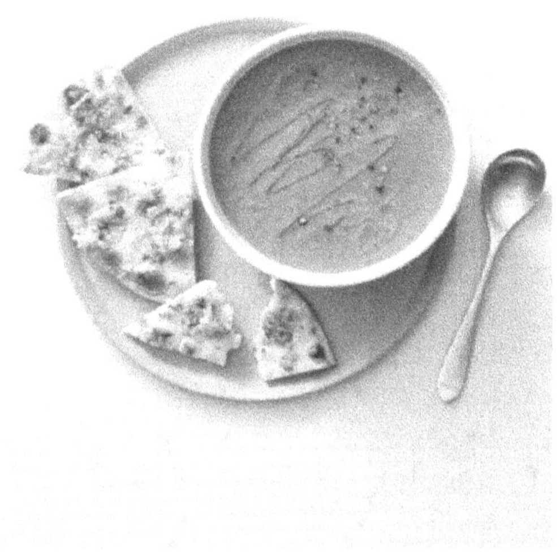

Cal/Serv	Yields	Prep Time	Total Time
325	4 servings	0 hours 10 mins	0 hours 25 mins

Ingredients

For Soup

- 2 tbsp. Olive oil
- 1 large onion
- 1 large red pepper (both chopped)
- 1/2 tsp. salt
- 2 cloves garlic
- 1 jalapeño
- 1-inch piece ginger
- 2 tsp. ground coriander
- 1 tsp. ground cumin

- 2 1/2 lb. Tomatoes (roughly chopped)
- 2 1/2 c. water
- 2 pocket less pitas

For Topping

- 1 tbsp. brown sugar
- 2 tbsp. butter or olive oil
- 2 tbsp. finely shredded unsweetened coconut
- 2 tbsp. cilantro

Instruction

- **Make soup:** Heat large Dutch oven on medium-low. Add olive oil, then onion, red pepper, and salt, and cook, covered, stirring occasionally, until tender, 8 to 10 minutes.
- Meanwhile, finely grate garlic, jalapeño, and ginger. Add to onion and cook, stirring, 1 minute. Stir in ground coriander and ground cumin and cook 1 minute.
- Add tomatoes and water; increase heat and simmer, partially covered, 10 minutes. While tomatoes are cooking, toast 2 pocketless pitas.
- Using immersion blender (or standard blender, in batches), puree soup until smooth.
- **Make topping:** Combine brown sugar in bowl with butter, finely shredded unsweetened coconut, and cilantro. Spread onto toasted pitas, then cut and serve with soup.

VEGAN QUESO

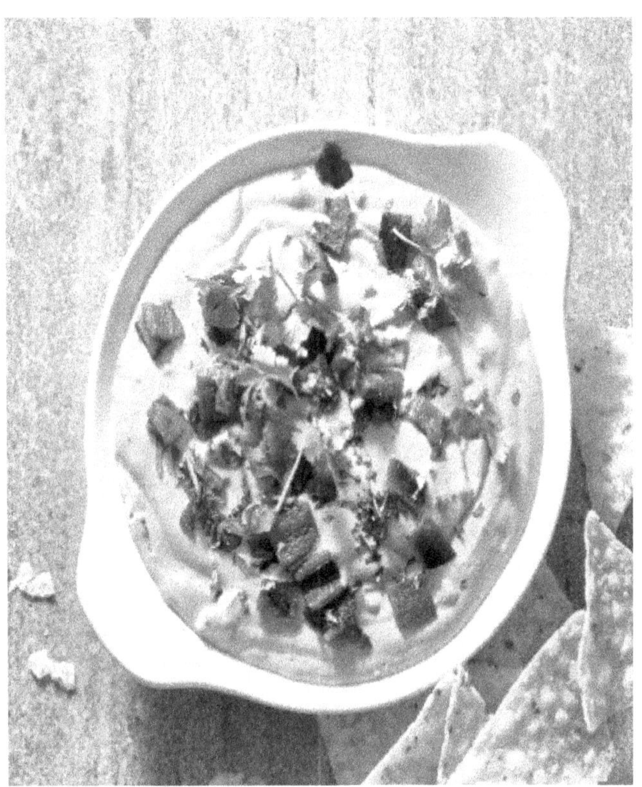

Yields	Total Time
8 servings	0 hours 45 mins

Ingredients

- 2 large poblano peppers, halved and seeded
- 1 tbsp. olive oil
- 2 cloves garlic, pressed
- 1 c. cashews
- 2 tsp. chili powder
- 1 tsp. ground cumin

- 1/2 tsp. ground coriander
- 1/2 tsp. ground turmeric
- Kosher salt and pepper
- 1/4 c. nutritional yeast
- Chopped cilantro and tortilla chips, for serving

Instruction

- Heat broiler. Arrange poblanos, cut sides down, on rimmed backing sheet and broil until charred, 3 to 5 minutes. Transfer to bowl, cover, and let sit 5 minutes. Use paper towel to remove skins, then cut peppers into ¼-inch pieces.
- Meanwhile, heat oil and garlic in small saucepan on medium until sizzling, about 1 minute. Remove from heat and stir in cashews, then spices and ½ teaspoon each salt and pepper. Add 1½ cups water and bring mixture to a boil. Reduce heat and simmer until cashews are tender, 10 to 12 minutes.
- Transfer mixture to blender, add nutritional yeast and ½ cup water, and puree until smooth.
- Return mixture to saucepan and cook, stirring occasionally, until thickened, 6 to 8 minutes. Fold in all but 2 tablespoons poblanos. Transfer to serving dish, top with remaining poblanos, and sprinkle with cilantro. Makes 2 cups. Serve with tortilla chips.

PRESSURE COOKER WINTER SQUASH AND LENTIL STEW

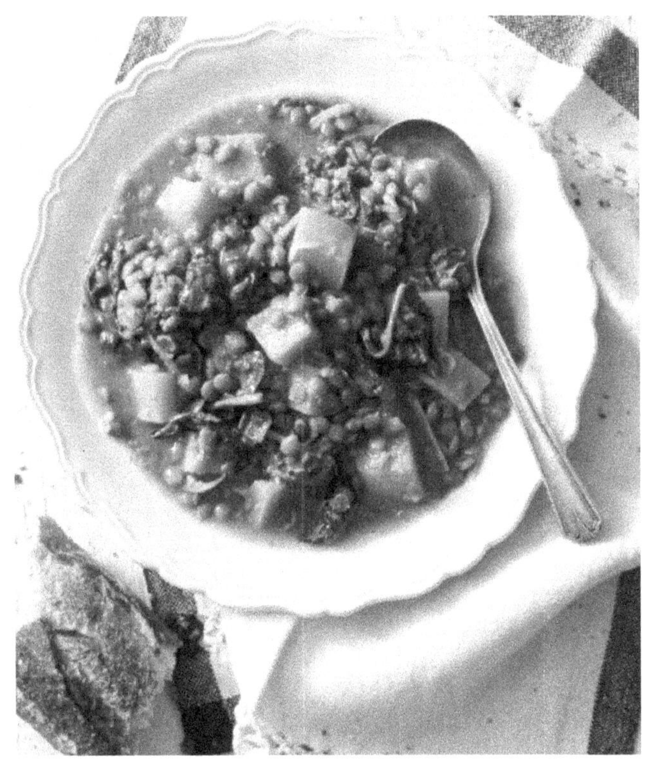

Yields	Prep Time	Total Time
6 servings	0 hours 15 mins	0 hours 35 mins

Ingredients

- 2 medium shallots, thinly sliced
- 1 tbsp. finely chopped peeled fresh ginger
- 1 tbsp. vegetable oil
- 1 tsp. ground coriander
- 1/2 tsp. ground cardamom

- 1 small butternut squash, peeled, seeded and cut into 1 1/2" chunks
- 1 lb. green lentils, picked over
- 6 c. chicken or vegetable broth
- 5 c. packed baby spinach
- 1 tbsp. cider vinegar

Instruction

- In pressure-cooker pot on medium, cook shallots and ginger in oil 5 minutes or until shallots are golden, stirring. Add coriander and cardamom; cook 1 minute, stirring. Add squash, lentils, broth and 1/4 teaspoon salt.
- Cover, lock and bring up to pressure on high. Reduce heat to medium-low. Cook 12 minutes. Release pressure by using quick-release function.
- Stir in spinach, vinegar and 1/2 teaspoon each of salt and pepper

EASY ROASTED VEGGIES AND TEMPEH BOWL RECIPE

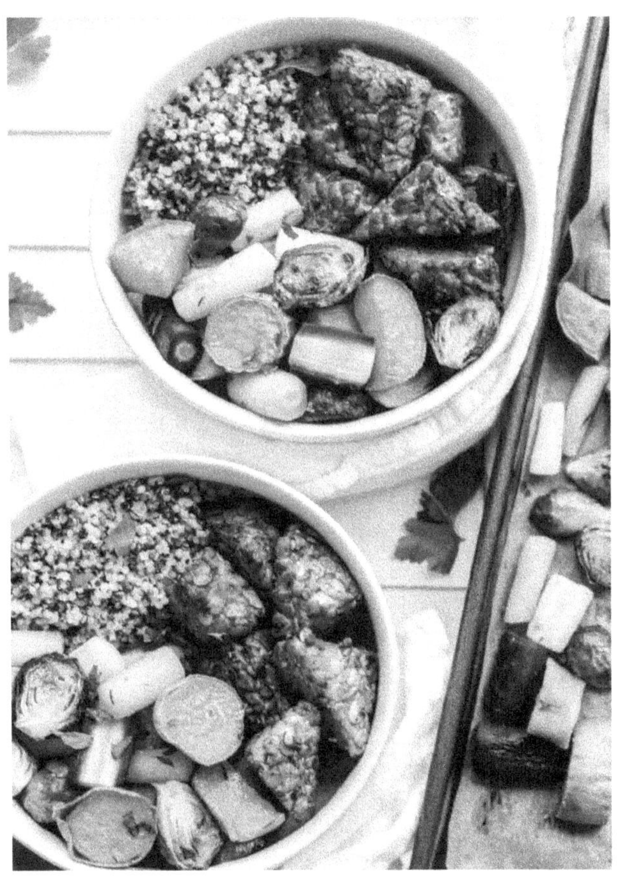

Yields	Total Time
1	0 hours 10 mins

Ingredients
- 1 c. baby spinach
- 1/2 c. shredded red cabbage

- 1/2 c. quinoa (recipe link in directions)
- 1 c. assorted roasted veggies
- 1 piece roasted tempeh (recipe link in directions)
- 2 tbsp. Chopped cilantro
- 1/4 tsp. toasted sesame oil
- Sliced radishes
- Lime wedge

Instruction

- Fill a bowl with baby spinach, shredded red cabbage, cooked quinoa, and assorted roasted veggies (we used ½ cup each tomatoes and broccoli).
- Top with roasted tempeh and chopped cilantro; drizzle with toasted sesame oil.
- Heat in microwave.
- Garnish with sliced radishes and a lime wedge.

RICOTTA PANCAKES.

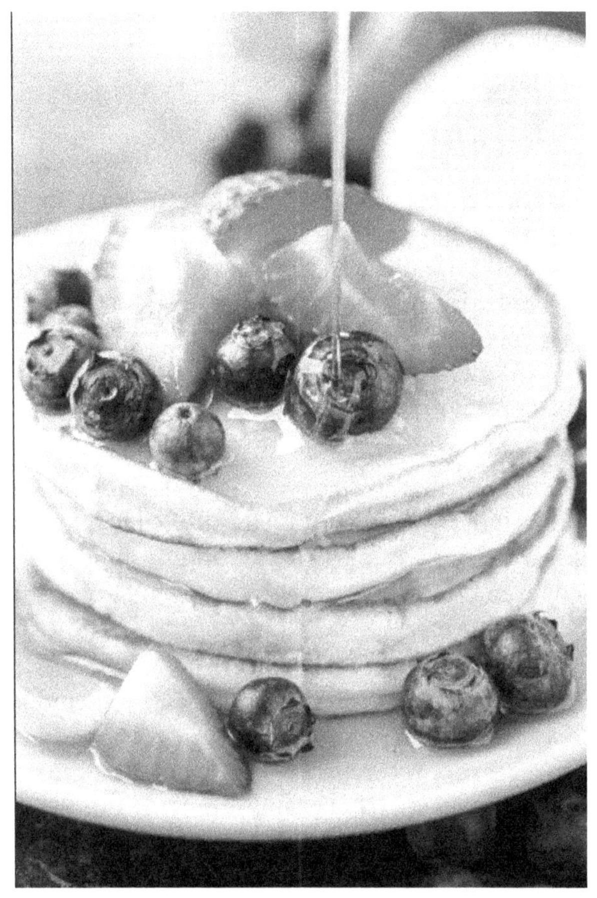

Cooking Time:

30 Mins

Server:

4

Ingredients

- 3/4 c. all-purpose flour, spooned and leveled
- 1/2 tsp. baking powder
- 1/2 tsp. kosher salt

- 1 c. whole-milk ricotta
- 3 large eggs, at room temperature and separated
- 1 tbsp. pure maple syrup
- 2 tsp. pure vanilla extract
- 3/4 c. whole milk
- Roasted Maple Rhubarb and Strawberries.

Instructions

- Set a wire rack in a baking sheet. Preheat oven to 200°F. Whisk together flour, baking powder, and salt in a bowl. Whisk together ricotta, egg yolks, maple syrup, and vanilla in a second bowl; whisk in milk. Fold dry ingredients into wet ingredients just until combined (mixture should be lumpy).
- Beat egg whites with an electric mixer on medium-high speed until stiff peaks form, 2 to 3 minutes. Gently fold egg whites into batter in two batches just until combined.
- Heat a large nonstick skillet over medium to medium-low heat. Drop batter by large spoonful (about 1/4 cup each) onto pan, gently spreading if necessary. Cook until bubbles begin to appear around edges and in centers, and bottoms are golden brown, 3 to 4 minutes. Gently flip. Cook, adjusting heat, if necessary, until golden brown on second side, 2 to 3 minutes.
- Transfer to prepared pan, cover loosely with foil, and keep warm in oven. Repeat with remaining batter. (If your pancakes stick, wipe skillet with 1 teaspoon canola oil before cooking the next batch.)
- Serve pancakes with Roasted Maple Rhubarb and Strawberries.

PINEAPPLE SMOOTHIE (PALEO OR VEGAN)

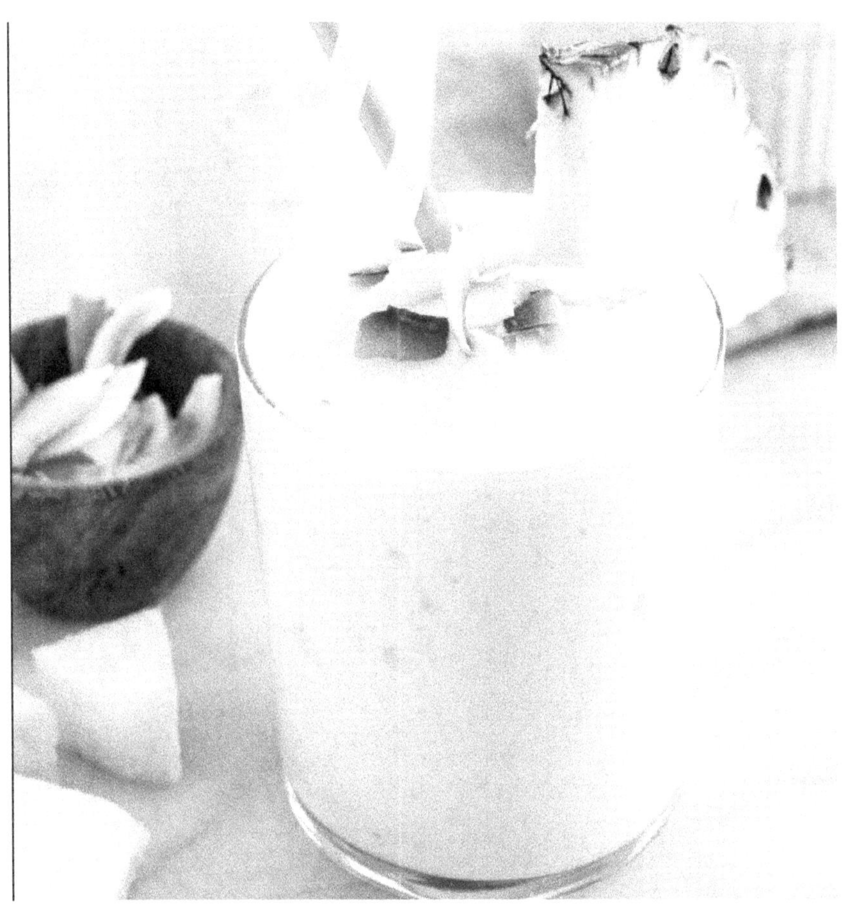

Prep Time:	Cook Time	Total Time:	Server
5 Minutes	0 Minutes	5 Minutes	4

Ingredients

- 2 cups frozen or fresh diced pineapple
- 1/2 ripe banana (fresh or frozen)

- 1 1/2 – 2 cups spinach or baby spinach
- 1 cup orange juice
- 1/2 tsp. vanilla extract
- 2 Scoops collagen protein (see notes for vegan options)
- Water as needed, to blend

ROASTED POTATO AND PEPPER HASH

This satisfying skillet recipe is easy and impressive.

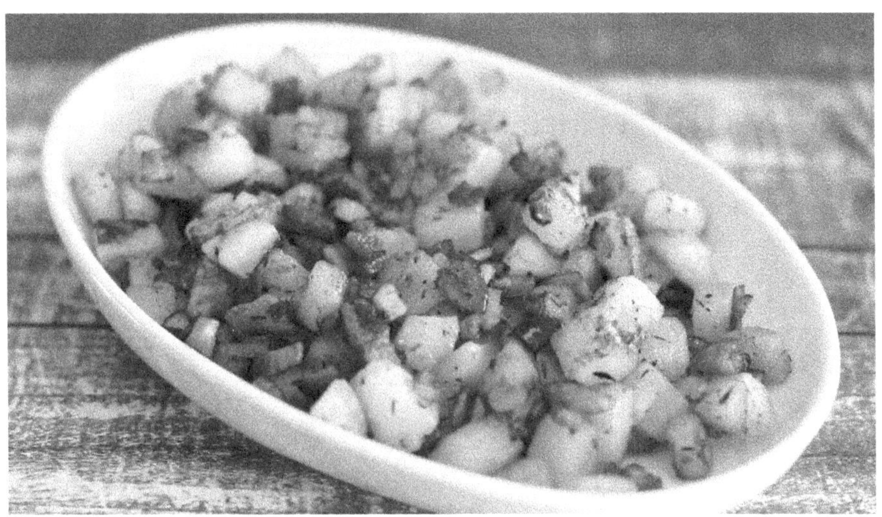

Cooking Time

30 Mins

Server

4

Ingredients

- 1 lb. Yukon gold potatoes, cut into 3/4-inch pieces
- 2 small bell peppers (1 red and 1 orange), cut into 3/4-inch pieces
- 1 red onion, cut into 1/2-inch pieces
- 4 cloves garlic, smashed
- 2 tbsp. olive oil
- Kosher salt and freshly ground black pepper
- 8 large eggs
- Chopped fresh flat-leaf parsley, for sprinkling.

Instructions

- Preheat oven to 425°F with oven rack 6 inches from heat. Toss together potatoes, peppers, onion, garlic, and oil in a 12-inch cast-iron skillet. Season with salt and pepper. Roast, stirring once, until potatoes are just tender and beginning to turn golden brown, 30 to 35 minutes.
- Remove skillet from oven and change oven setting to broil. Make 8 small wells in vegetable mixture, and carefully crack an egg into each. Broil to desired doneness, 4 to 6 minutes for a runny yolk. Sprinkle with parsley just before serving.

FLUFFY VEGAN PANCAKES.

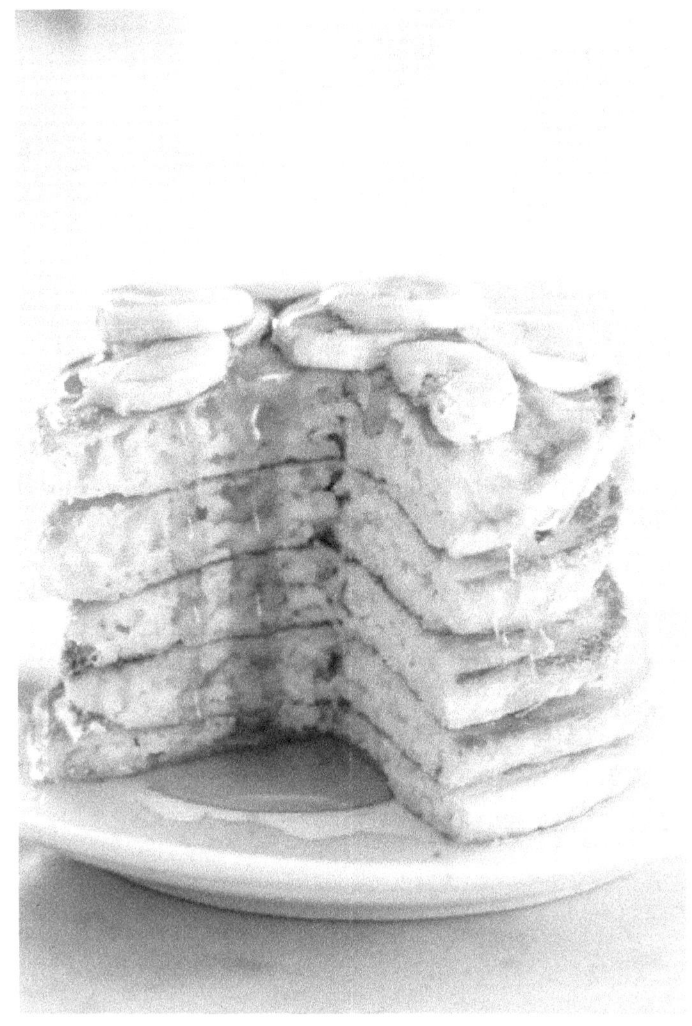

Prep Time	Cook Time	Total Time	Server
5 minutes	15 minutes	20 minutes	2-4

Ingredients

- 1 c. all-purpose flour
- 1 tbsp. granulated sugar
- 1 tbsp. baking powder
- 1/4 tsp. salt
- 1 c. almond milk (or any other non-dairy milk)
- 2 tbsp. coconut oil
- Vegetable or coconut oil, for frying
- Maple syrup, for serving
- Fresh fruit, for serving (optional).

Instructions

- In a large bowl, whisk together flour, sugar, baking powder, and salt. Add almond milk and coconut oil and mix until smooth.
- In a large skillet over medium low heat, heat oil. Using a 1/4 cup measure, pour batter into pan. Cook 2 to 3 minutes, and flip when you see bubbles forming around the edges of the pancakes. Cook 2 to 3 minutes more on the opposite side, until golden. (If making a large, preheat oven to 200° and place prepared pancakes on baking sheet in oven.)
- When all batter has been used, serve with maple syrup and toppings of your choice.

BUCKWHEAT PORRIDGE

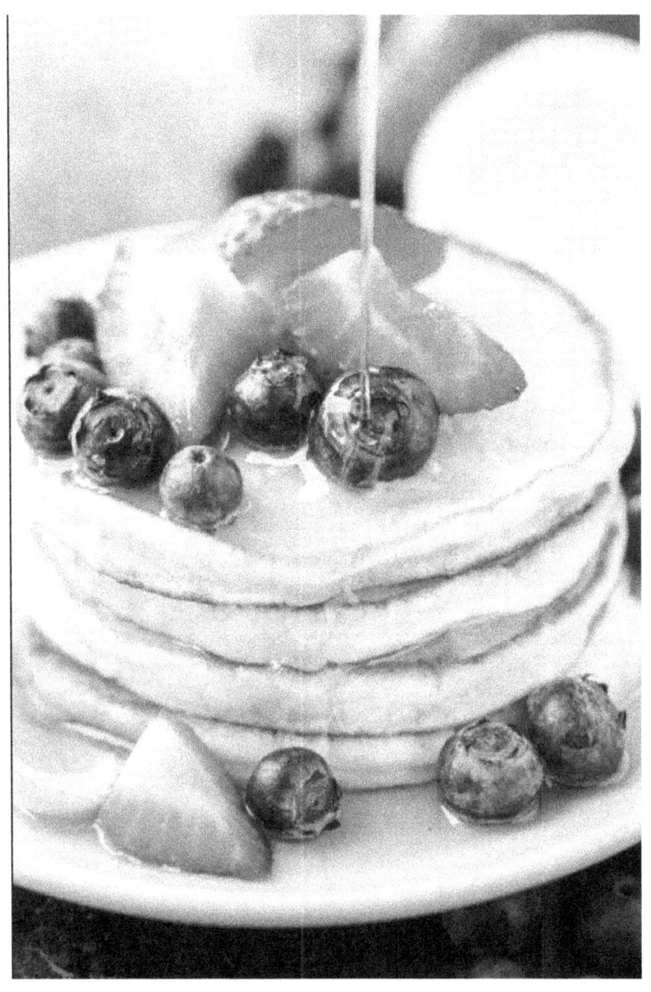

Cooking Time

20 Mins

Server

4

Ingredients

- 2 cups buckwheat groats

- 2 cups coconut milk
- 2 cups water
- 3 tablespoons maple syrup, or sweetener of choice
- 1 teaspoon vanilla
- 1 dash nutmeg, (optional)
- 1 dash cinnamon, or cardamom (optional)
- 1/4 teaspoon salt

Instructions

- Place the pan on medium heat and add water and coconut milk.
- Rinse the Buckwheat and add it to the saucepan.
- Once the mixture starts boiling, reduce the heat.
- Let it simmer for a minute or two.
- Add vanilla extracts, cinnamon, or cardamom powder.
- Cover the pot and let it cook for 10 minutes.
- Turn off the heat after 10 minutes but keep the lid on.
- Remove the lid after 5 minutes.
- Pour the porridge into the bowl and garnish it with fresh fruit of your choice.
- Drizzle maple syrup on top and enjoy.

EASY VEGAN LEMON POPPY SEED MUFFINS.

Soft, fluffy vegan lemon poppy seed muffins that are perfect for snacking!

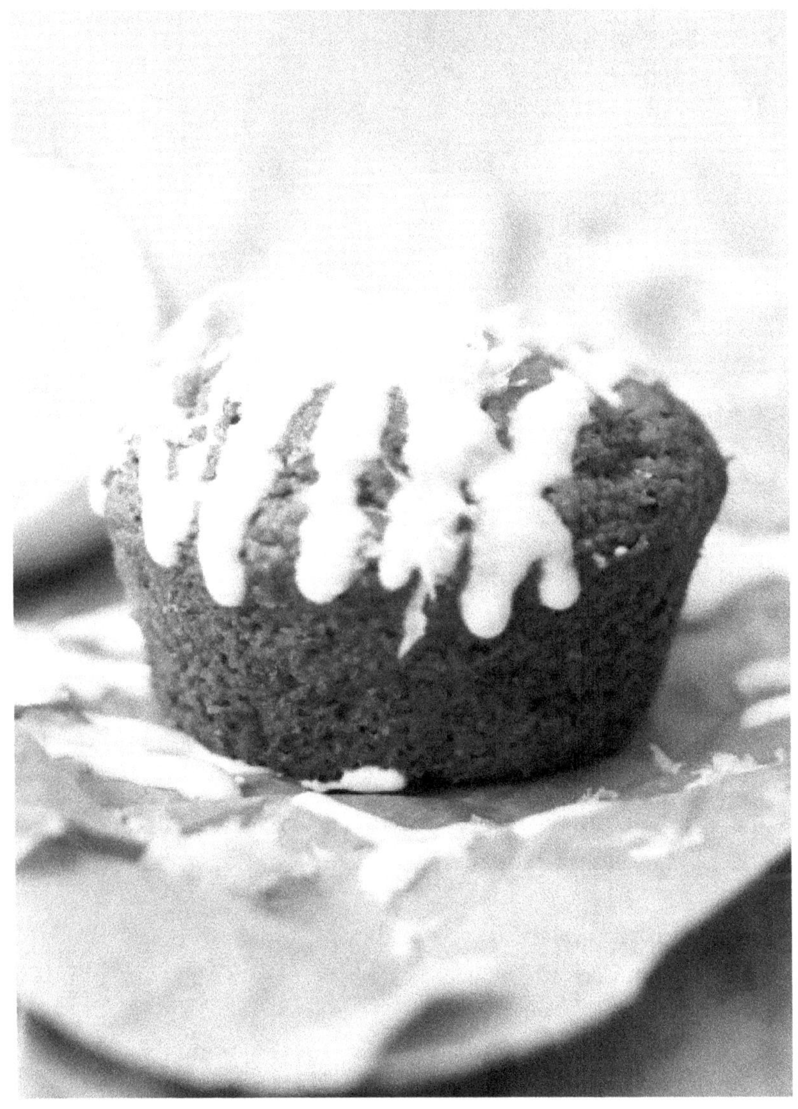

Prep Time	**Cook Time**	**Total Time:**	**Server**
12 minutes	17 minutes	29 minutes	10

Ingredients

- 2 tbsp lemon zest
- 1 tbsp poppy seeds
- Dry Ingredients
- 1½ cups all-purpose flour
- ½ cup white sugar
- ½ tsp salt
- 2 tsp baking powder
- Wet Ingredients
- ⅓ cup melted vegan butter
- ⅓ cup plain unsweetened applesauce
- ⅔ cups unsweetened almond milk + 2 tsp apple cider vinegar
- ½ tsp lemon extract
- ¼ cup unsweetened almond milk
- Icing
- 1 cup organic powdered sugar
- 4 tsp lemon juice

Instructions

- Preheat oven to 400°
- Measure out ⅔ cups of unsweetened almond milk and add 2 tsp apple cider vinegar. Set aside.
- In a large mixing bowl, mix together the dry ingredients.
- Add in the wet ingredients and whisk together to combine. Batter may still be a little lumpy.
- Gently mix in the lemon zest and poppy seeds.
- Evenly disperse the batter into your muffin pan using a ¼ measuring cup.
- Place in preheated oven and bake for 17 minutes or until they bounce back up after gently touching them.

- While the muffins are baking, whisk together the ingredients for the icing. Set aside.
- Once the muffins are finished baking, set them aside and allow to cool completely.

VEGAN STRAWBERRY POP TARTS

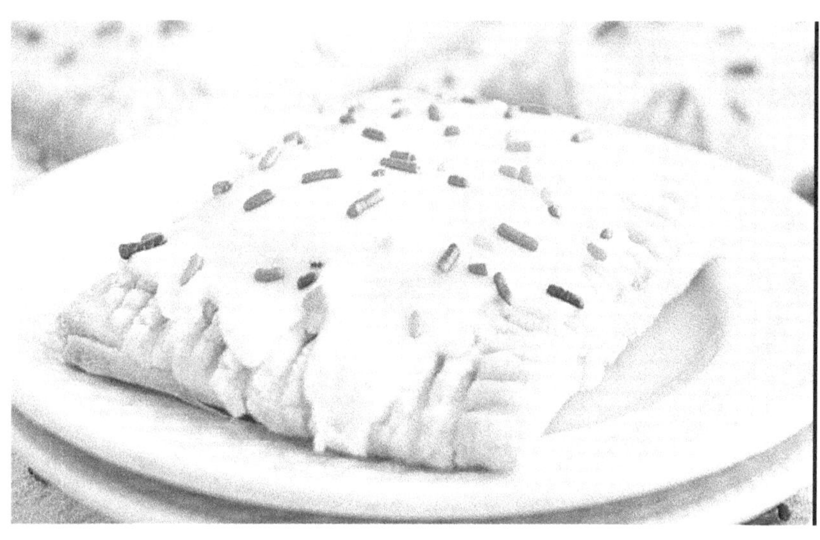

Prep Time:	Cook Time	Total Time:	Server
30 Minutes	30 Minutes	1 Hr 30 Mins	4

Ingredients

- For the Strawberry Filling
- 2 cups strawberries, stems removed
- 1/2 cup water, divided
- 1/4 cup vegan cane sugar
- 2 tbsp cornstarch (sub for arrowroot powder)
- For the vegan crust
- 3 cups flour (can use GF – see post)
- 1/2 tsp salt
- 1/2 tsp sugar
- 18 tbsp vegan shortening
- 1/2 cup unsweetened dairy free milk, + more for brushing
- 1/4 tsp vanilla extract
- For the Icing

- 2 cups powdered sugar
- 4-6 tsp water
- 1/4 tsp vanilla
- chopped freeze dried strawberries or sprinkles

Instructions

- For the Strawberry Filling
- Remove stems from strawberries.
- Add berries, 1/4 cup water, and sugar to a sauce pot over medium heat. Stir together. Then, bring to a boil.
- Lower heat and mash the berries with a potato masher. Let reduce for 8-10 minutes.
- In a small bowl add remaining 1/4 cup water and cornstarch. Whisk together to dissolve.
- Remove berry mixture from heat and add cornstarch mixture immediately. Stir constantly while adding.
- Let cool completely before adding to dough.
- For the vegan crust
- In a large bowl, add the flour, salt, and sugar. Stir together with a fork.
- Cut vegan shortening into tablespoon size cubes and then using a fork combine together until crumbly.
- Pour in milk and vanilla.
- Stir until combined.
- Use hands to form a dough.
- Lay a piece of parchment paper down and sprinkle with flour. Lay dough down and sprinkle with a touch of flour on top.
- Roll out dough into an 18×24 inch rectangle.
- Tip: If you don't have a lot of counter space, split dough in half and roll out each piece into a 9×12 inch rectangle.
- Cut the dough vertically from the longest side every 3 inches. You should end up with 8 strips of dough.
- *If doing the 2 9×12 rectangles, cut each piece into 4 strips.
- Lightly brush the dough with vegan milk.
- Preheat oven to 425 degrees.
- Once strawberry filling has cooled completely, fill the lower 4 inches of dough with mixture, about 1-2 tablespoons. Leave 1/2 inch between each side.

- Fold the top half of the dough over on top of the bottom.
- Firmly press them together trying not to leave any air pockets.
- Use a fork and press along all the edges.
- Place on a baking sheet lined with parchment paper.
- Brush the tops with more vegan milk.
- Bake for 20-30 minutes or until lightly golden brown on top and around edges.
- Place on a cooling rack and let cool completely.
- Make the icing by adding powdered sugar to a bowl and whisk in a teaspoon of water at a time until slightly runny.
- Add in the vanilla and whisk again.
- Dip the tops of the pop tarts into the icing or drizzle on top.
- Add chopped freeze dried strawberries or sprinkles on top if desired.
- Serve or store in an air tight container – room temperature for 1-2 or 7 days in the fridge. Can freeze for up to 6 months.

VEGAN PUMPKIN WAFFLES

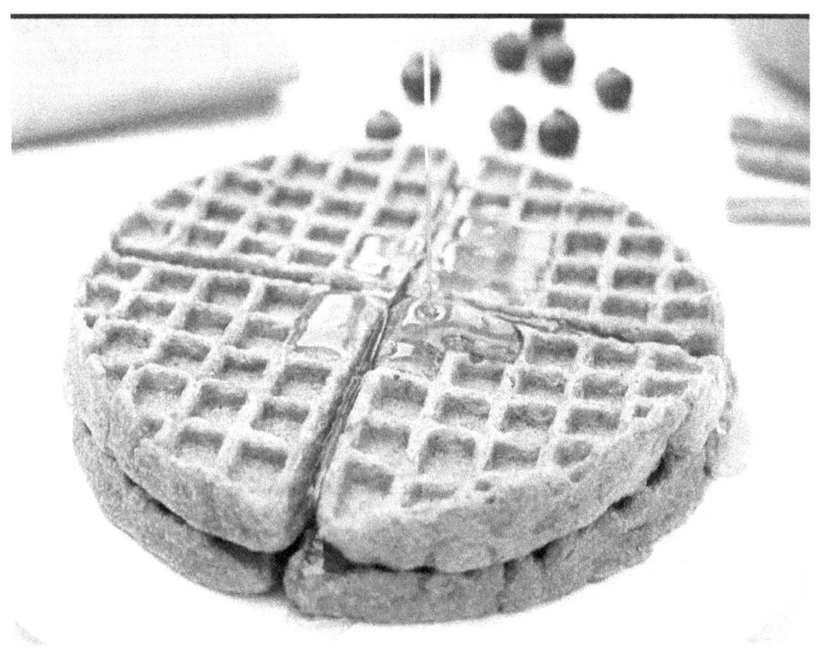

Prep Time	Cooking Time	Total Time:	Serving
10 Minutes	10 Minutes	20 Minutes	8

These Vegan Pumpkin Waffles are full of pumpkin spice goodness and are the perfect Fall weekend breakfast! Crispy on the outside and fluffy on the inside. 1 Bowl.

Ingredients

- 15 ounces canned pumpkin
- 1/4 cup melted coconut oil
- 2 cups soy milk
- 1/4 cup granulated sugar

- 2 1/4 cups all-purpose flour
- 2 teaspoons baking powder
- 1/2 teaspoon baking soda
- 1/2 teaspoon salt
- 2 teaspoons cinnamon
- 1/2 teaspoon ground ginger
- 1/4 teaspoon ground nutmeg.

Instructions

- Preheat your waffle iron.
- In a large bowl, whisk together the canned pumpkin, oil, soy milk and sugar until smooth.
- Add the flour to the bowl with the wet ingredients, then sprinkle on top of the flour the baking powder, baking soda, salt and spices. Mix with a large spoon until just combined. The batter should be fairly thick, not too runny. If it's runny, add a little more flour. If it gets too thick, add a little water.
- Spray waffle iron well with oil (unless your waffle iron is non-stick). Pour the recommended amount of batter onto hot waffle iron, and cook until the waffle is golden brown on both sides.
- Serve immediately, or keep in a warm oven (200 degrees F) until ready to serve. Top with vegan whipped cream, vegan butter, maple syrup and anything else you desire!

VEGAN FRENCH TOAST CASSEROLE

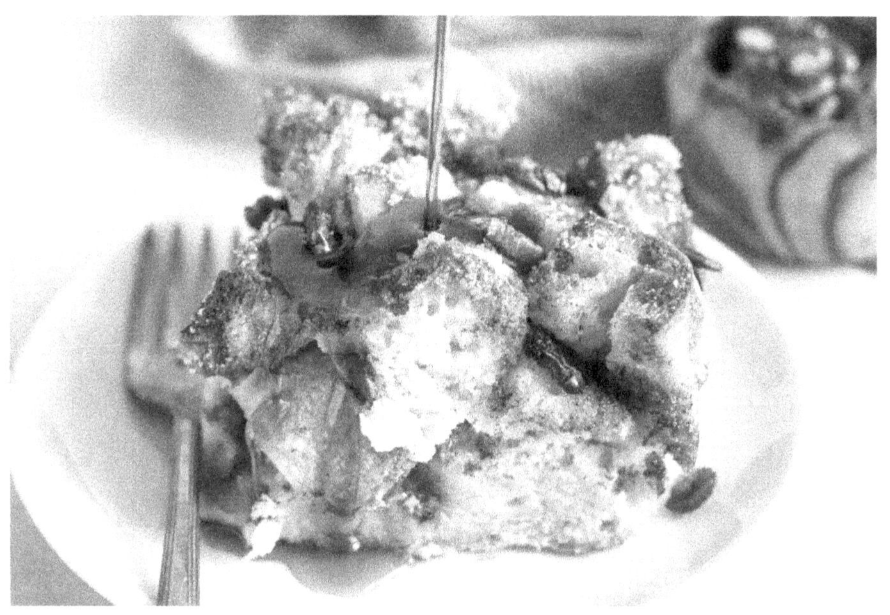

Prep Time:	Cooking Time	Total Time:	Servings
10 Minutes	50 Minutes	60 Minutes	8

Ingredients

- 1-day old large loaf (14-16 ounces) French or sourdough bread*, cut into 1-inch cubes (about 10 cups)
- 12 ounces silken tofu
- (1) 13.5-ounce can full fat coconut milk
- 2 tablespoons cornstarch
- 1/2 cup granulated sugar
- 1 tablespoon pure vanilla extract
- 1 teaspoon ground cinnamon
- 1/4 teaspoon salt

Instructions

- Prepare the bread: Cut the bread into 1 inch cubes. I do this by first slicing the loaf, then cutting into smaller cubes. Lightly grease a 9 by 13 inch casserole dish, and add the bread cubes to it.
- Make the custard: In a blender, add the silken tofu (drained of water if needed), coconut milk, cornstarch, sugar, vanilla, cinnamon and salt. Blend until smooth.
- Pour the custard over the bread cubes. Using your hands, press the bread down into the custard a few times, until the bread is soaked in it. Cover and place in the refrigerator for 8-12 hours. You can bake it immediately if you prefer.
- In the morning, preheat the oven to 350 degrees F.
- Make the topping: In a small bowl, combine the brown sugar, flour and cinnamon. Then cut the vegan butter in with a fork or your fingers. Sprinkle this over the top of the casserole.
- Bake, uncovered, for 40-50 minutes, until golden brown on top and cooked throughout.

VEGAN BLUEBERRY AND COCONUT MUFFINS

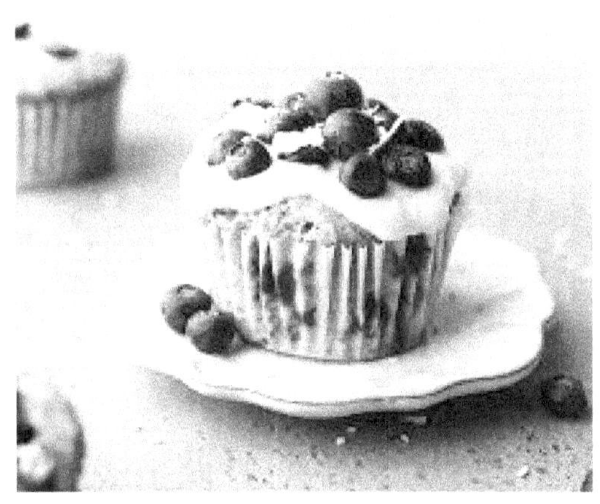

Prep Time	Cooking Time	Total Time:	Serving
15 Minutes	25 Minutes	40 Minutes	6

Ingredients

- 75g vegan butter
- 140g light brown sugar
- 2 flax eggs*
- 110g coconut yoghurt
- 60ml vegan milk (coconut/almond/oat)
- 1.5 tbsp lemon juice
- 2 tsp vanilla essence
- 180g plain flour
- 2 tsp baking powder
- 1 tsp baking soda
- 6 tbsp desiccated coconut
- 150g blueberries

- Optional Topping
- Coconut yoghurt
- Blueberries

Instructions

- Preheat the oven to 180C/350F.
- In a large bowl mix the butter and sugar until light and fluffy.
- Next add the flax eggs, coconut yoghurt, milk, lemon juice, vanilla and stir.
- Then sieve and add the flour, baking powder and baking soda. Fold in with the wet ingredients and then add the desiccated coconut and blueberries until combined.
- Spoon into 6 large muffin cases. Place into the oven for 25 minutes. Check they are ready by inserting a skewer, if it comes out clean, they are ready. If not, leave for a few more minutes.
- Leave to cool in the tin for 5-10 minutes before transferring to a cooling rack.
- Enjoy straight away or keep in an air tight container for 2-3 days. I like to serve mine with some extra coconut yoghurt and blueberries on top.

COCONUT & BANANA PANCAKES

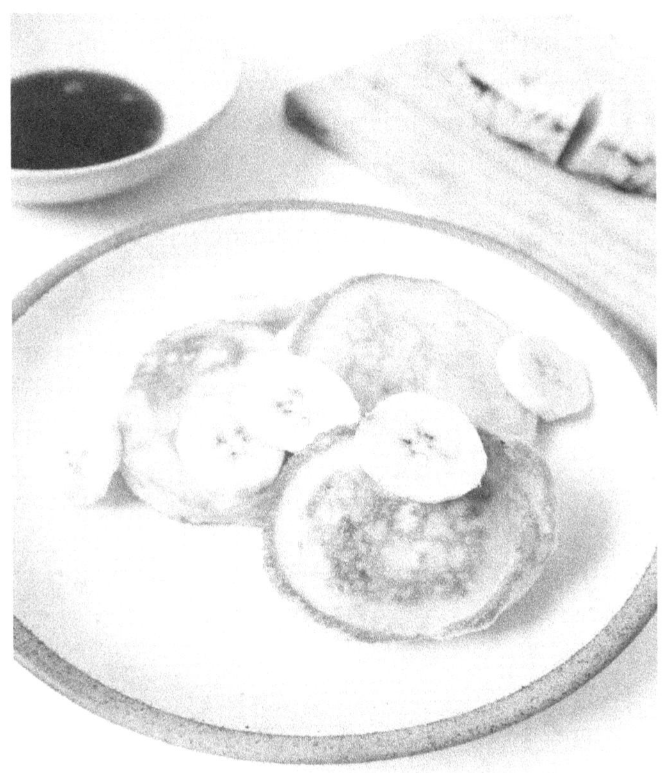

Cooking Time	Yields	Prep Time	Total Time
15 Mins	4 Servings	10 Mins	25 Mins

Ingredients:

- Plain flour   (1 ½ gram)
- Baking Powder   (2tbsp)
- Golden caster sugar   (3tbsp)
- Coconut milk   (2 cups)
- Oil of your choice   (for frying)

- Thinly sliced banana   (1-2 only)
- Passion Fruits   (only 2)

Instructions:

- Take a bowl and sift the flour and baking powder into it.
- Now stir in 2 tbsp of the sugar and a pinch of salt.
- Then put the coconut milk into a bowl, mix any fat that has separated, and then measure out 1 cup into a jug.
- Whizz everything with a blender to make a smooth batter.
- Now take a shallow frying pan and heat it.
- Use 2 tbsp. of batter to make each pancake, frying only two at a time more than two makes it difficult to flip them.
- Then push 4-5 slices of banana into each pancake and cook until the edges look dry and bubbles start to pop on the surface.
- Now turn them over carefully and cook the other sides for a minute.
- Meanwhile, take a small pan and pour the remaining coconut milk and sugar into it.
- Then add a pinch of salt and simmer until the mixture thickens to the consistency of single cream, and use this as a sauce for pancakes.

VEGAN BREAKFAST MUFFINS

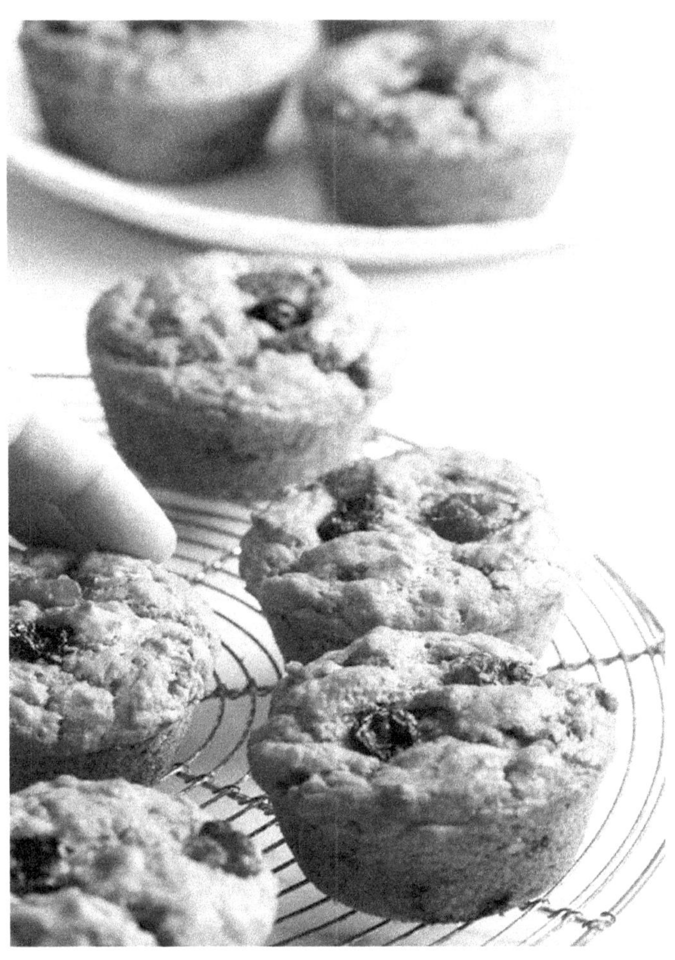

Cooking Time	Yields	Prep Time	Total Time
25 Mins	4 Servings	25 Mins	50 Mins

Ingredients:

- Muesli mix (9 tsp)
- Light brown soft sugar (3 tsp)
- Plain flour (1 ½ cup)

- Baking powder   (1 tbsp)
- Sweetened almond milk   (1 ½ cup)
- Peeled and grated apple   (only 2)
- Oil of your choice   (2 tbsp)
- Nut butter   (3 tbsp)
- Demerara sugar   (4 tbsp)

Instructions:

- Gather all ingredients.
- Heat the oven to 200C/180C fan/gas 6 and line a muffin tin with cases.
- Now put 100g muesli with light brown sugar, baking powder, and flour in a bowl and mix well.
- Take a jug and combine the milk, apple, oil, and 2 tbsp nut butter into it, then stir into the dry mixture.
- Now divide equally between the cases.
- Then mix the remaining muesli with the demerara sugar, remaining nut butter, and the pecans, and spoon over the muffins.
- Now bake it for 25-30 minutes or until the muffins are risen and golden.
- Will keep for two to three days in an airtight container or freeze for one month.
- Refresh in the oven before serving.

VEGAN FRENCH TOAST

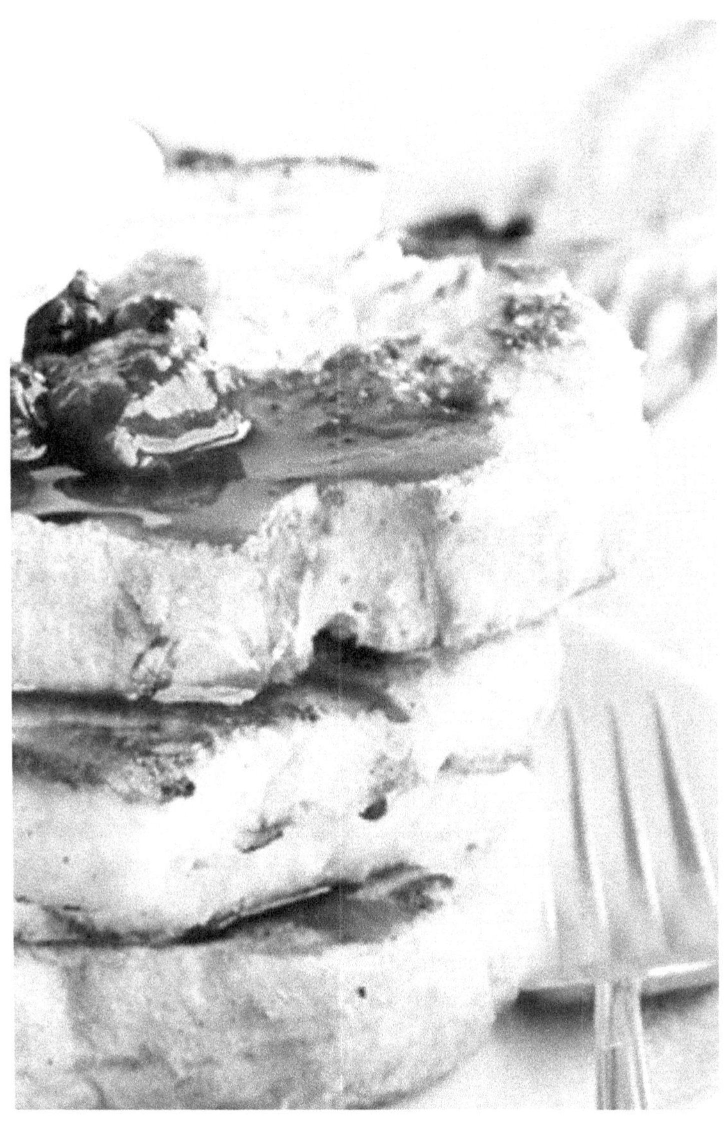

Cooking Time	Yields	Prep Time	Total Time
25 Mins	4 Servings	20 Mins	40 Mins

Ingredients:

- Maple syrup   (1 tbsp)
- Blueberries   (1 cup)
- Gram flour   (2 tbsp)
- Ground almonds   (2 tbsp)
- Cinnamon   (2 tbsp)
- Oat milk or rice milk   (1/2 cup)
- Golden caster sugar   (1 tbsp)
- Vanilla extract   (1 tbsp)
- Thick white bread (6 slices)
- Oil of your choice   (for frying)
- Icing sugar   (for dusting)

Instructions:

- Firstly, Gather all ingredients.
- Now take a saucepan and put maple syrup and blueberries into it and heat it until the berries start to pop and release their juice.
- Then set them to one side in the pan.
- Now take a shallow bowl and whisk the flour, cinnamon, milk, almonds, and vanilla together into the bowl.
- Heat a little oil in a frying pan.
- Then dip a slice of bread into the milk mixture, shake off any excess.
- Now fry the bread on both sides until it browns and crisps at the edges.
- Remember; keep the slices warm in a low oven as you cook the rest.
- Your breakfast is ready.
- Serve it with the blueberries spooned over and dust with icing sugar.

MAPLE OATMEAL

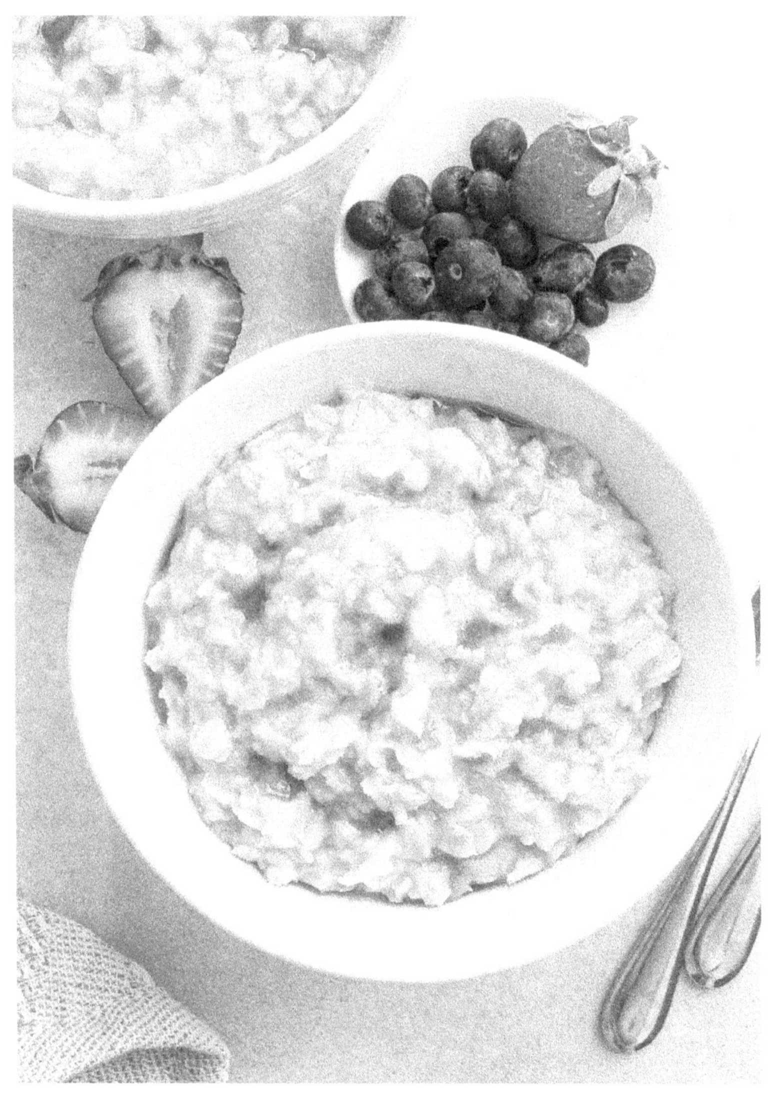

Cooking Time	Yields	Prep Time	Total Time
20 Mins	5 Servings	20 Mins	50 Mins

Ingredients:

- Maple syrup   (1 tbsp)
- Berries   (1/2 cup)
- Ground almonds   (2 tbsp)
- Cinnamon   (1/4 tbsp)
- Almond milk   (1/2 cup)
- Vanilla extract   (1/4 tbsp)
- Oats   (1/2 cup)
- Chia seeds   (1 tsp)
- Salt to taste

Instructions:

- Bring the water, almond milk, vanilla and salt to a low boil on the stovetop.
  Add oats and chia seed, and reduce heat to simmer.
- Simmer on low for 3-5 minutes, and remove from heat.
- Let sit 5 minutes to thicken.
- Stir in cinnamon and maple syrup, and top with berries if desired.
- Serve immediately.

RASPBERRY RIPPLE CHIA PUDDING

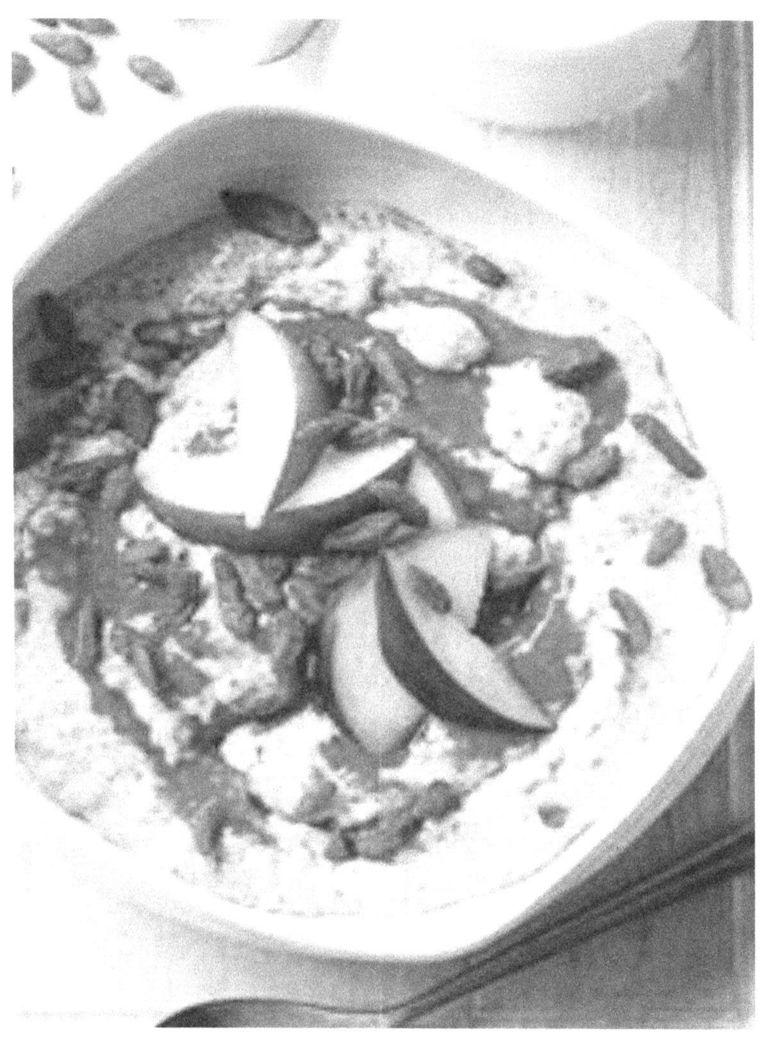

Ingredients:

- White chia seeds   (3 tsp)
- Coconut drinking milk   (1/2 cup)
- Slices of nectarine or peach   (only 1)
- Goji berries   (2 tbsp)

For the raspberries puree:

- Raspberries   (1/2 cup)
- Lemon juice   (1 tbsp)
- Maple syrup   (2 tbsp)

Instructions:

- Firstly, Gather all ingredients.
- Now take two serving bowls and divide the chia seeds and coconut milk between these bowls and stir well.
- Then leave to soak for 5 minutes, and stirring occasionally until the seeds swell and thicken when stirred.
- After that, take a small food processor and combine the puree ingredients into it, or blitz with a hand blender.
- Now swirl a spoonful into each bowl.
- Then arrange the peach slices or nectarine on top and scatter with the goji berries.
- Will keep it in the fridge for one day.
- Add the toppings just before serving.

BLACK BEANS & AVOCADO TOAST

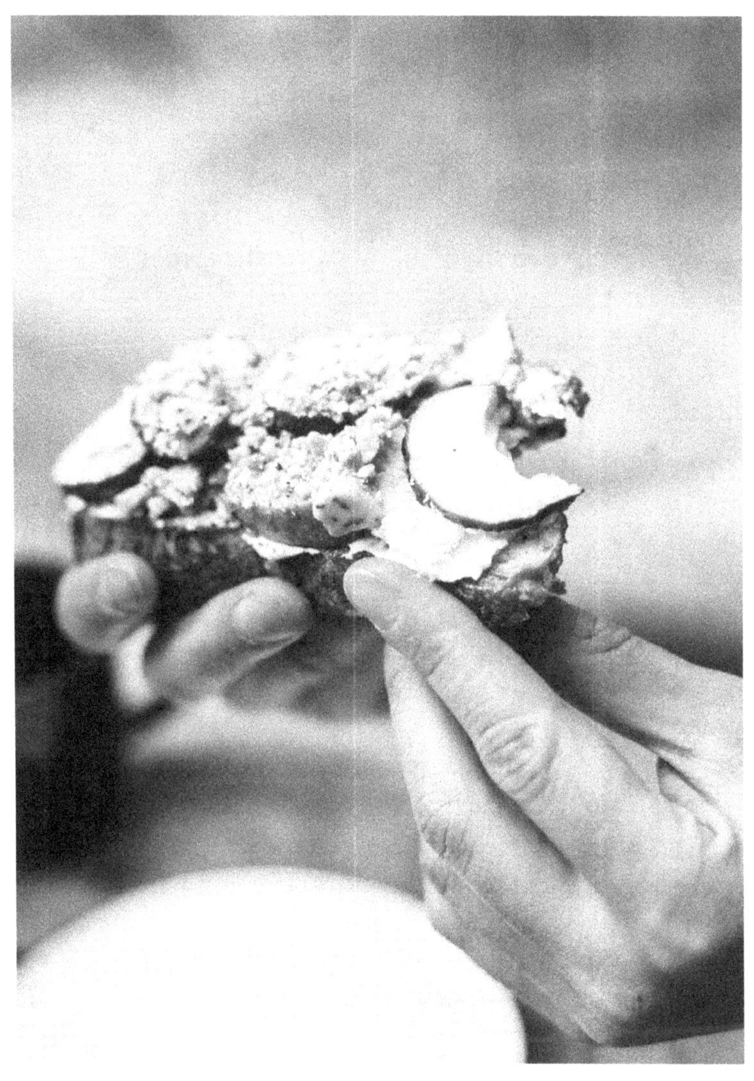

Cooking Time	Yields	Prep Time	Total Time
10 Mins	5 Servings	20 Mins	30 Mins

Ingredients:

- Cherry tomatoes   (2cups)
- Finely chopped onion   (only 1)
- Lime juice   (1/2 tbsp)
- Oil of your choice   (4 tbsp)
- Crushed garlic cloves   (only 2)
- Ground cumin   (1 tbsp)
- Chipotle paste   (2 tbsp)
- Drained black beans   (3 cups)
- Chopped coriander   (A small bunch)
- Sliced bread   (4 slices)
- Finely sliced avocado   (only 1)

Instructions:

- Firstly, gather all ingredients.
- Now mix the tomatoes, 12 tbsp lime juice, ½ onion, and 1 tbsp oil and set aside.
- Then fry the remaining onion in 2 tbsp oil until it starts to soften.
- Add the garlic and fry it for 1 minute, then add the cumin and chipotle and stir until fragrant.
- Now tip in the beans and splash of water, stir and cook gently until heated through.
- Stir in most of the tomato mixture and cook for 1 minute.
- Season well and add most of the coriander.
- Now toast the bread and drizzle with the remaining 1 tbsp oil.
- Take plates and put a slice on each plate and pile some beans on top.
- Now take avocado slices and arrange them on top.
- Then sprinkle with the remaining tomato mixture and coriander leaves to serve.

SWEET POTATO FRIES

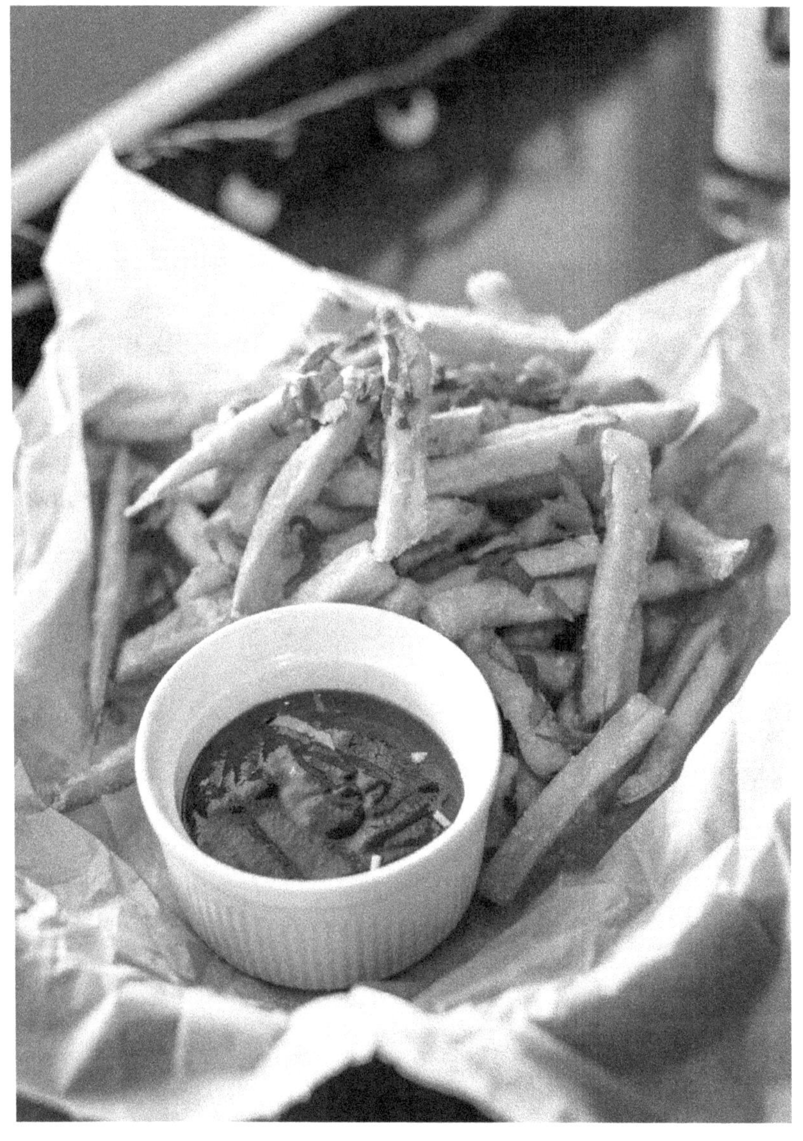

Cooking Time   Yields   Prep Time   Total Time

0 Mins   4 Servings   5 Mins   5 Mins

Ingredients:

- Sweet potatoes   (2 pounds)
- Oil of your choice   (2 tsp)
- Paprika   (1 tsp)
- Salt   (1 tsp)
- Black pepper   (1/2 tsp)

Instructions:

- Preheat the oven to 400 degrees.
- Peel and cut sweet potatoes into sticks and toss with oil.
- Mix the spices, salt, and pepper in a bowl and toss with sweet potatoes. Spread on baking sheet.
- Bake for about 15 minutes until brown and crispy.
- Serve with tomato sauce or any other sauce you like and enjoy.

VEGAN BANANA FRENCH TOAST WITH CARAMELIZED BANANAS

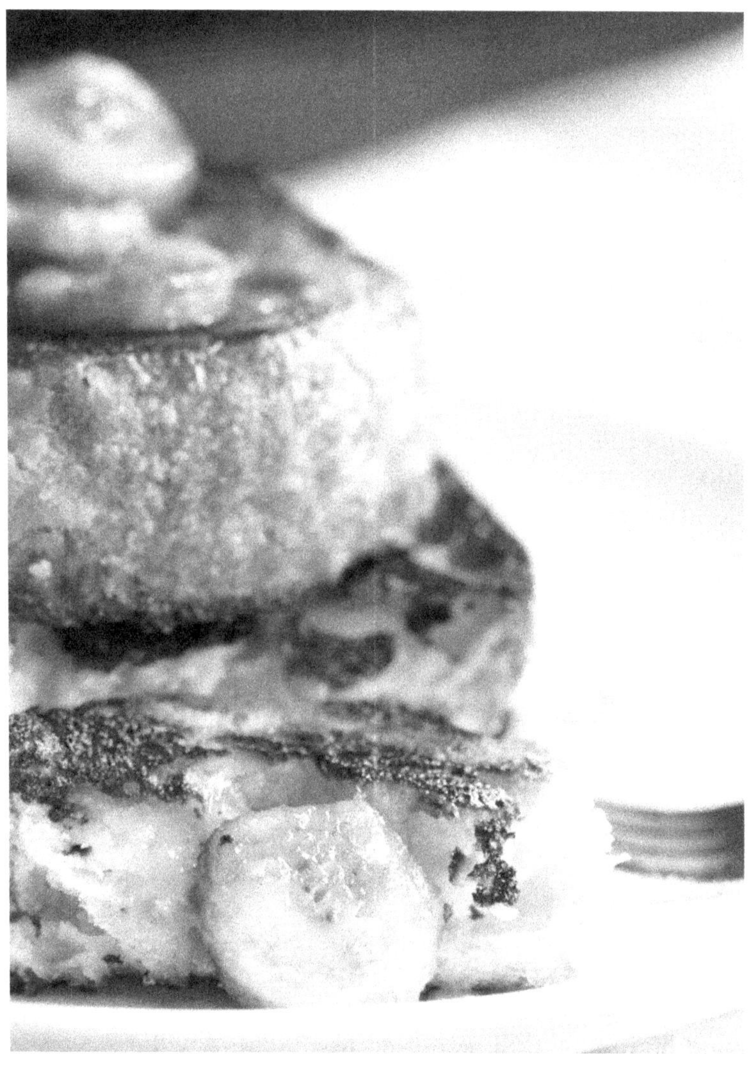

Cooking Time	Yields	Prep Time	Total Time
25 Mins	4 Servings	10 Mins	35 Mins

Ingredients:

- Sliced 1loaf day-old rustic bread

For toast batter:

- Small to medium banana   (only 1)
- Almond milk   (1/2 cup)
- Maple syrup   (2tbsp)
- White flour   (2tbsp)
- Vanilla extract   (1/2tbsp)
- Oil   (1tbsp)
- Nutmeg   (1/4tbsp)
- A very good pinch of black pepper & salt

For caramelized banana:

- Sliced banana   (2 ripe)
- Coconut sugar or brown sugar   (2tbsp)
- Nondairy milk   (2tbsp)
- A good pinch of nutmeg and cinnamon

Instructions:

- Firstly gather all ingredients, then blend everything under French toast batter and transfer to a shallow bowl.
- Now take a frying pan and heat the oil into it over medium heat. Then place bread slice in the batter for 2 seconds, then flip and soak for 2seconds more.
- Remove the batter and let the excess fall off for 2-3seconds. Place in the hot frying pan.
- Now cook for 4-6minutes per side. Cook at medium-low heat if your stove runs hot.
- Cook the batter well and caramelize the banana in it but not burn it. If the French toast is not done, the bread will not release from the pan easily. Let it cook for 1minute more or so. Then flip and cook the other side.
- Now add a helping of the caramelized bananas, maple syrup, vegan butter, and some fresh fruit and serve immediately on a serving plate.

Caramelized bananas:

- Combine banana slices, non-dairy milk, nutmeg, sugar, and a pinch of salt in a frying pan over medium heat. Cook about 6minutes or until the mixture thickens.
- Stir occasionally. Make a double batch of these to serve on the side or over oatmeal

VEGAN FRY-UP

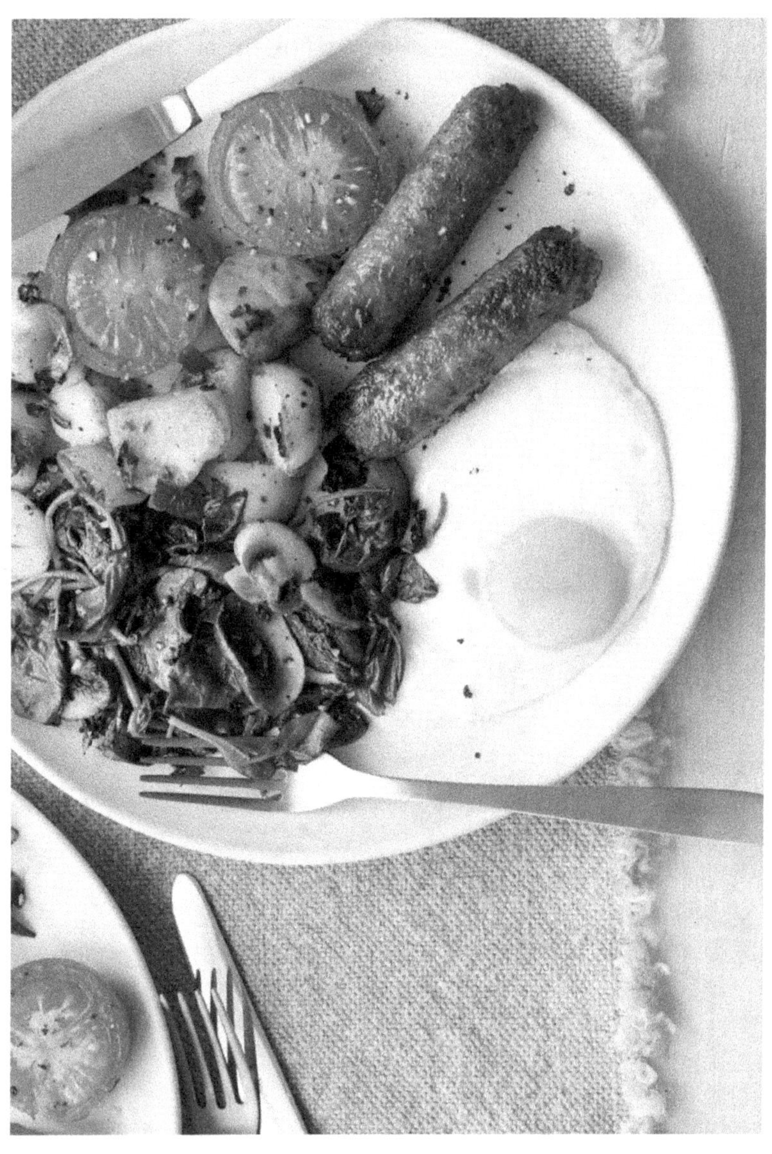

Cooking Time	Yields	Prep Time	Total Time
30 Mins	4 Servings	15 Mins	45 Mins

Ingredients:

- Unpeeled potato   (1 large)
- Bell peppers   (1 ½ tbsp)
- Onion   (only 1)

For the tomatoes and mushrooms:

- 14 Cherry tomatoes
- Oil of your choice
- Maple syrup   (2 tbsp)
- Sauce   (1 tbsp)
- Smoked paprika   (1/4 tbsp)
- Portobello mushroom   (1 large) sliced

For the scrambled tempeh:

- Silken tempeh   (3 cups)
- Nutritional yeast   (2 tbsp)
- Turmeric   (1/2 tbsp)
- Crushed garlic clove   (only 1)

To serve:

- 4 vegan sausages
- 1 x 200g can baked beans

Instructions:

- Cook the whole potato in a large pan of water, boil for 10minutes, and then drain and let it cool.
- Peel the skin of the potato away then coarsely grate. Mix it with bell peppers and season well.
- Then set it aside in the fridge until needed.
- Now heat oven to 200C/180C fan/gas 6. Then take a baking tray and put the cherry tomatoes into it, drizzle with 2 tbsp oil, season and bake for 30 minutes or until the skin has blistered and started to char.
- After that cook the beans and sausages by following the instructions on the pack so they are ready to serve at the same time as the scrambled tempeh.

- Meanwhile, take a large bowl and mix the maple syrup, sauce, and ¼ tbsp. smoked paprika together into it, then add the sliced mushroom and toss to coat in the mixture.

- Leave to stand while you take a non-stick frying pan pour 2 tbsp oil into it and bring it up to medium-high heat.

- Now fry the mushroom until just starting to turn golden but not charred. Scoop onto a plate and keep warm until serving.

- Pour 1 tbsp oil into the frying pan and add spoonful of the potato mixture you should get about 4. Then fry it for 3-4inutes each side then drain onto kitchen paper.

- Crumble the tempeh into your frying pan and scatter over the remaining ingredients and a good pinch of pepper and salt.

- You can add a splash more oil if the pan looks a little dry. Then fry for 3-4minutes or until the tempeh is broken into pieces, well coated in the seasoning, and hot through.

- Now take two plates and divide everything between these plates and serve with a hot mug of tea made using almond milk.

BANANA BAKED OATMEAL

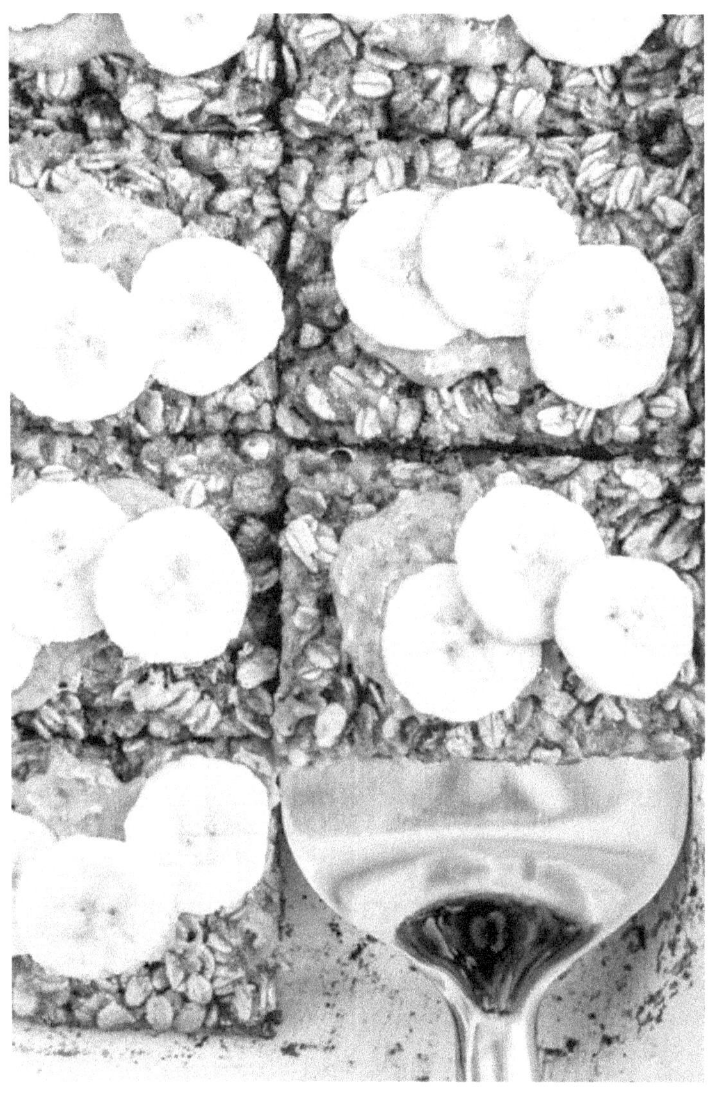

Cooking Time	Yields	Prep Time	Total Time
45 Mins	4 Servings	15 Mins	60 Mins

Ingredients:

- Rolled oats   (2 cups)
- Pecan pieces   (1/2 cup)
- Cinnamon   (1 ½ tbsp.)
- Allspice   (1/2tbsp)
- Kosher salt   (1/2tbsp)
- Mashed banana   (3/4 cup)
- Almond or oat milk   (1 ¾ cups)
- Pure maple syrup   (1/4 cup)
- Pure vanilla extract   (1tbsp)
- Banana slices   (to serve)
- Almond or peanut butter (to serve)

Instructions:

- Gather all ingredients, and preheat the oven to 375F.
- Now take a frying pan and grease with oil. Then mix the rolled oats, allspice, baking powder, cinnamon, kosher salt, and pecan pieces in a medium bowl.
- Add the dries to the prepared pan.
- Now whisk together the mashed bananas, maple syrup, vanilla, and milk in the same bowl. Then drizzle the milk mixture over the oats.
- Stirring lightly with a fork to make everything gets evenly incorporated.
- Now bake for 40-45 minutes or until the top is nicely golden and the oat mixture has set. Then remove from the oven and let it cool for at least 10minutes.
- Spread the top with almond butter or peanut butter before serving and top with banana slices.
- You can store leftovers in a refrigerator for up to 1 week: reheat in a 300-degree oven or microwave until warm.